# BLADDER PROBLEMS

# BLADDER PROBLEMS

## A Complete Self-Help Guide

Rosy Reynolds

Thorsons
An Imprint of HarperCollins*Publishers*
77-85 Fulham Palace Road,
Hammersmith, London W6 8JB

Published by Thorsons 1991
1   3   5   7   9   10   8   6   4   2

A CIP catalogue record for this book
is available from the British Library.

ISBN 0 7225 2508 7

Typeset by Harper Phototypesetters Limited,
Northampton, England
Printed in Great Britain by
HarperCollinsManufacturing, Glasgow

# CONTENTS

# Note to the Reader

Throughout this book doctors are referred to as 'he'. This is purely for the sake of convenience, because no single term yet exists to denote 'he/she'. Therefore 'he', in this context, should be taken to mean 'he or she'.

# ACKNOWLEDGEMENTS

I would like to thank the following people who read and made helpful comments on the manuscript: Chris Benness MRCOG MRACOG, Ranju Beswick MRPharmS, Linda Cardozo MD MRCOG, Karen Dixon, Stephanie Mumby, Gill Stenning SRN SCM ADM and especially Paul G. Carter MB ChB FRCS(Ed) and Nick Dixon PhD BM BCh.

Thanks also to Bristol University Library for allowing me to use their facilities.

For Duncan, who made it necessary,
and Dave, who made it possible.

# Chapter 1

# INTRODUCTION

Incontinence is not yet a respectable disorder. While sinus trouble and heart surgery are fit to be discussed at the dinner table, and cystitis and hysterectomy are acceptable coffee break conversation, incontinence is almost unmentionable. It might just surface as a problem for a friend who looks after an elderly relative, but a healthy young woman who admits publicly to a problem of bladder control risks shocking her companions at the very least.

Illness, of course, has no respect for social nicety: we may proscribe incontinence from our conversation but we cannot so easily exclude it from our lives. In fact 30 per cent or more of women between 25 and 65 sometimes lose urine unintentionally; for 10 per cent or more this is a regular occurrence. There are also many women whose bladders demand to be emptied with intense urgency or extreme frequency. They may never actually leak but their lives are disrupted by the behaviour of their bladders. In addition, it is estimated that over half the women in most western industrialized countries suffer from cystitis at some time in their lives. If you have a bladder problem, however isolated you may feel, you are in company with millions of others!

Cystitis is in a different category from the troubles covered in detail in this book. It occurs as separate attacks rather than as an ongoing problem and, although a bout of cystitis is very unpleasant, it is not

9

seen as a disgraceful secret. It is not too difficult to approach a doctor for help or to find advice in books, so the nuisance it causes can be kept within limits.

The other bladder problems can cause distress out of all proportion to their physical significance. The need to reach a toilet quickly, or the need to use a pad to soak up leaked urine, might be trivial in itself but there is the feeling that people will ridicule you for having to visit the toilet so often. There is the fear that they will be disgusted to notice a damp patch or a clinging smell. There is the dread of the humiliation if you were to be caught short in public, and there is the social isolation that these fears can produce. What really matters is not the loss of urine but the loss of friends, activities and, worst of all, self-esteem.

Far too many women have put up with the restrictions placed upon them by their urinary ailments for far too long. Some find their condition so shameful that they are too embarrassed to confess their difficulties to a doctor. Many others see no point in consulting a doctor because they believe that nothing can be done. This attitude of resignation, which flourishes while incontinence remains taboo, is misplaced. Most bladder problems can be alleviated, many can be cured. None need be accepted without a fight.

It is over 40 years since Kegel introduced a program of pelvic muscle exercise, and nearly 20 years since Frewen described a scheme of bladder training. Both of these methods are suitable as self-help treatments and together they offer the probability of improvement to the majority of women with bladder troubles. There are further medical techniques available for use in cases where these simpler methods are not appropriate.

It is absurd, considering how commonplace and how remediable most bladder problems are, that we should allow them to cause such unhappiness. Why be ashamed of a disorder in your urinary system? You would not worry in that way over a torn ligament or a stomach ulcer. Why let it shake your self-confidence? The fault is in your bladder, not in your brain; you are still the same competent, capable, worthwhile person. Why feel helpless? There is plenty to be done, and in most cases you can do it yourself.

Why bear it when you might beat it?

# Chapter 2

# WHAT'S THE PROBLEM?

When I was a teacher, like many other teachers, I preferred my pupils not to know my first name. I invented apparently practical reasons for this but really it was no more than a modern manifestation of the 'primitive' belief that a name carries power. To know your enemy's name gives you the advantage over him; to let him know yours is sheer foolhardiness.

In the battle for full bladder control, it is an advantage to know the medical term for your particular problem. In practical terms, you can then choose the most appropriate self-help treatment. In primitive terms, you know your enemy's name.

## Stress Incontinence

In stress incontinence you lose urine accidentally as a result of physical exertion; it has nothing at all to do with mental or emotional stress. The events which most typically cause leakage are coughing, sneezing or laughing. Running, jumping and similar athletic activities are also major culprits. In more severe cases gentler movements such as walking, getting up from a chair or even simply turning over in bed can cause urine loss.

Typically, the amount of urine lost each time is small but, if you suffer severely, a succession of small leaks combine to give you the depressing feeling of being always wet. Usually, you are aware of the leakage but there is no feeling that you need or want to empty your bladder. If you lose larger amounts of urine and only ever as a result of laughter, your problem may be giggle incontinence (see below) rather than stress incontinence.

When you say you have stress incontinence you are simply describing a symptom. You are not saying anything about the cause. Very often the cause is 'sphincter incompetence' (see below), and if this is the sole cause a doctor or urologist will call the condition 'genuine stress incontinence'. This is a rather unfortunate name because it means that doctors classify the other cases of stress incontinence as 'not genuine', and patients can misunderstand them as meaning that there is no real physical problem. In fact they only mean that there is some cause additional to, or other than, a weak sphincter. If you leak as a result of physical activity, you have stress incontinence and nobody will suggest otherwise although they may find other names to describe its cause.

# Urgency and Urge Incontinence

For people with healthy bladder control, the question of where and when to empty the bladder is mainly a matter of convenience. As their bladders fill, they become aware of a mild desire to void. If the time or place is inconvenient, the desire can safely be ignored and will usually pass off. Only when the bladder has been ignored repeatedly and allowed to fill to capacity does the urge to empty it become irresistible.

If you have urgency, the desire to empty your bladder comes on suddenly and is overwhelmingly strong right from the start. You have an immediate urgent need to reach a toilet, and probably a substantial fear of losing urine on the way. If your fears are realized and you leak before reaching the toilet, that is urge incontinence.

Urgency and urge incontinence are so closely related that the distinction between them may depend on trivial practicalities, such as the stiffness of your trouser zip. They differ from stress incontinence because they always involve a pressing desire to empty the bladder. With urgency, you may never actually lose any urine but the need always to be within easy reach of a toilet and the fear of being caught short can cripple your social life just as surely as actual incontinence.

# Frequency and Nocturia

Frequency means emptying your bladder more frequently than normal. It is usually defined as urinating seven or more times during the waking day, which corresponds to an average interval of about two and a half hours between trips to the toilet.

There are a variety of causes for frequency, some trivial, some not, and a variety of reactions to it. You may be perfectly happy to empty your bladder eight times in a day but it is undeniably disruptive if you cannot last more than half an hour between toilet visits.

Nocturia literally means urinating during the night but, medically, it does not include bedwetting and many doctors feel that a single toilet trip a night is too commonplace to count, particularly in older people. A sedentary lifestyle allows fluid to pool in the legs during the day; this fluid is excreted when it returns to the central circulation on lying down at night. Also, older people tend to sleep more lightly and so are more easily disturbed by their bladders filling. In active younger people, nocturia is closely related to daytime frequency and hardly ever occurs on its own.

If you are going to the toilet for something to do because you cannot sleep, your difficulty is really insomnia rather than nocturia.

# Bedwetting

The correct medical name for this is nocturnal enuresis but bedwetting describes the condition equally accurately. There is a complete coordinated emptying of the bladder. The only difference between this and an intentional emptying is that you remain asleep. Some people dream that they are using a toilet; others have no awareness of their bladder's misbehaviour until they wake in the morning to a wet bed. It is a particularly frustrating problem to have because, since you are not even awake at the time, there seems to be nothing you can do about it. Luckily you can take action during the day which will affect your bladder's behaviour at night.

# Giggle Incontinence (Giggle Micturition)

'You should have seen it, I almost wet myself' is an expression universal amongst teenage girls to describe their enjoyment in those hugely, enormously, hysterically funny events which happen so often in healthy energetic young lives. For those who must leave out the 'almost', the fun has an untimely and abrupt end.

In giggle incontinence, extreme mirth provokes the bladder to start emptying itself. If you are very quick and have very good control of the muscles which stop urine flow you may be able to limit the amount of urine lost, but it is difficult to gain control while you are laughing hysterically and your bladder may empty completely. It is especially annoying that situations funny enough to produce a leak almost always arise when you are in company with your friends so it is a particularly difficult problem to keep private.

# Dribbling Incontinence

If you lose urine the whole time in a steady dribble, see your doctor. It could be due to an injury which has left an abnormal hole (fistula) connecting some part of your urinary system to the outside. Alternatively, something may have gone wrong with your bladder's emptying mechanism so that it is being filled beyond the normal limits until the pressure inside is raised so much that urine is forced out constantly (overflow incontinence). Either way, you need medical help.

Severe stress incontinence can make you constantly wet but it differs from dribbling incontinence because the urine is not lost steadily but in separate spurts, each one caused by some slight movement.

# Cystitis/Urethral Syndrome

These names are vague. They do not cover a single condition with a single cause and the corresponding symptoms are variable. The most consistent are a stinging or burning pain when you pass water and a feeling of need to urinate very frequently. Chapter 11 describes the variety of symptoms in more detail and explains the basic self-help routine.

# Dysuria

This term means pain when you urinate. If it fits the description for cystitis in Chapter 11 you can try self-help for a couple of days, but seek medical advice if it carries on any longer.

# Haematuria

Haematuria is blood in your urine. This can be a rather alarming symptom but it is usually less momentous than it first appears. However, you must see a doctor as it can sometimes be a sign of something seriously amiss. Unless you are losing a great deal of blood you need not call him out at midnight for this but, even if the bleeding seems to have stopped, make an appointment within a day or two. You will need to supply a midstream urine specimen to be tested for infection and traces of blood.

# After-Dribble

This is properly called post-micturition dribble and it is the loss of a small amount of urine several seconds after you have finished emptying your bladder, usually after replacing your clothes. If it is your only symptom it is not medically significant but it can be still be very embarrassing.

In women, the likely cause is urine collecting in the vagina so the remedy is simple. Have a piece of toilet paper in place to catch the drips and keep yourself over the toilet while you stand up and allow the urine to escape. (In men, the dribble is of urine left in the 'U-bend' of the longer urethra; it can be squeezed into the penis to be emptied in the usual way by pressing firmly upwards on the perineum a little way forward of the anus and drawing the fingers forward.)

# Terminal Dribble

Terminal dribble means that when you empty your bladder, the last part of the urine leaves in an annoyingly slow dribble or in fits and starts instead of in a single steady stream with a definite end. This difficulty usually affects men of middle age and over, and is most often caused by enlargement of the prostate gland.

# Hesitancy, Slow Stream

Hesitancy means difficulty in starting the stream of urine and slow stream, naturally enough, means that the flow is meagre even when it has started. Like terminal dribble, these can be early signs of prostate enlargement in men.

# Unstable Bladder (Detrusor Instability)

An unstable bladder contracts as if to expel its contents at unsuitable times and against the wishes of its owner. The contractions may happen for no apparent reason at all, or as an inappropriate reaction to filling, or in response to such diverse stimuli as the sound of running water, a cough or a sudden movement. Unstable bladders can play a part in stress incontinence, but they are particularly associated with urgency and urge incontinence. You may suspect that bladder instability is a factor in your stress incontinence if the leak follows the cough with a short delay, if there is no leak until the third or fourth in a series of coughs or if the volume of urine lost is large.

The only way to diagnose detrusor instability for certain is to place pressure-measuring devices in the bladder and in either the vagina or rectum and measure the pressure in both places simultaneously. In this way a doctor can distinguish between contractions of the bladder muscle (which affect only the bladder pressure) and abdominal movements (which affect both). This technique is only available after referral to a specialist urological unit.

# Sphincter Incompetence

If the sphincter mechanism which should prevent urine leakage is not strong enough to stand up to the pressures put on it by normal physical activity, it is said to be incompetent. It is a shame that 'incompetence' carries such strong overtones of bungling, blame and personal responsibility in everyday language because, medically speaking, it is only a description of a physical fact. When stress incontinence occurs without any other symptoms, sphincter incompetence is the usual cause.

To prove that the sphincter mechanism is incompetent it must be shown to allow urine leakage in the absence of active bladder contractions so the diagnosis again involves the elaborate technique of simultaneous pressure recording, this time to rule out unstable bladder activity.

From a self-help standpoint you cannot be absolutely certain whether you have an unstable bladder or an incompetent sphincter or a bit of both but you will do well enough by choosing your treatment on the basis of your symptoms. The core of the treatment for stress incontinence in Chapter 7 is pelvic floor exercise to strengthen the muscles which support and control the bladder outlet, but there are also elements intended to help re-train an unruly bladder. The approach to frequency, urgency and urge incontinence in Chapter 8 is an intensive course of bladder training which should relieve your symptoms whether or not bladder instability is at the root of them. Bladder training is also relevant if you suffer from bedwetting, and sections from both programs are useful for giggle incontinence.

# Chapter 3

# SHOULD YOU SEE A DOCTOR?

'But why don't they complain?' my doctor friend asked, genuinely puzzled. This was off-duty, a conversation between friends at a party, and he was surprised to hear how widespread a problem stress incontinence is. 'I don't think it is that common' he had objected when I complained that, for such a common problem, absurdly little is taught about it to women at risk. Once convinced that solid research results did not bear out the impression he had gained from the small number of patients arriving at his practice, he was perplexed. 'Why don't they complain?'

Perhaps the biggest barrier is not knowing what the doctor could possibly do. Obviously, if he can do nothing there is no point in seeing him, and plenty of women believe (wrongly) that nothing can be done to relieve their difficulties. 'That's the price of childbearing' they say resignedly, or 'I've always had a weak bladder — I suppose it's just a woman's problem' or, saddest of all, 'What can you expect at my age?' At the other extreme, they may be afraid of the (imagined) treatment itself and dread that they may be subjected to intrusive examinations or taken into hospital for surgery.

Then there is the belief that they shouldn't waste the doctor's time. 'Yes,' they agree 'the bladder problem is an awful nuisance but I can live with it and the doctor has more important things to deal with.' There are many women who will put up with a remarkable degree of discomfort and inconvenience rather than be seen to be complaining while there are others worse off.

Finally, there is the embarrassment. We are generally coy about our excretory functions in our society, even when they are working normally; for many women it is difficult just to find the words to explain what has gone wrong. But it is not only a question of words, it is a question of feelings. Bladder problems, and incontinence in particular, have an extraordinary capacity to make women feel bad about themselves — dirty, ashamed, worthless — and knowing that the feelings are ill-founded does not make them go away. Women may be so afraid that the doctor will despise them, or that other people may find out their secret, that they prefer to struggle on alone rather than take the risk of seeking help.

Is it worth trying to overcome these objections to seeing a doctor? Naturally it depends on how great the benefits of seeking medical advice might be, so what are the possible advantages?

First of all, very occasionally, a bladder problem like incontinence can be a symptom of something more seriously wrong. If your doctor suspects this he will be able to arrange appropriate tests or treatment for the underlying illness. On the rare occasions when some serious disorder is at the root of the trouble it is clearly important to find out about it. Very much more often, the bladder problem is just what it seems and your doctor will be able to reassure you that there is nothing more serious to worry about.

Secondly, there are some bladder problems which are treated more effectively by a doctor than by self-help. For example, long-term low-grade bladder infections sometimes produce confusing symptoms of urgency or mild stress incontinence rather than the classic symptoms of cystitis. You might not suspect an infection but the doctor could identify it by testing a urine specimen and treat it with an antibiotic. It is particularly worthwhile seeing your doctor if your bladder symptoms started in connection with the menopause or while taking medicines for some other condition, because there is a good chance that he will be able to help immediately in these cases too. You should also let your doctor know immediately if your difficulties began soon after a surgical operation.

Thirdly, if yours is a supportive and sympathetic doctor, you will feel better simply from having talked about the problem. If you have kept it secret for years it is a great relief to find that you can tell someone without their being disgusted or even surprised. The doctor may also be able to encourage you in starting and sticking to a self-help program. In this book I can only talk in general terms about what applies to most people with urge incontinence or bedwetting or whatever, and you may still doubt whether it applies to you, so the support of a doctor who knows you personally could be very valuable.

Finally, many bladder problems can be cured and most can be alleviated. There are extremely few which cannot be effectively treated. Even if bladder function cannot be returned to normal (following a spinal injury, perhaps, or in a disease like multiple sclerosis), there are techniques for managing the problem, and a number of very good aids and appliances have been devised to solve some of the practical difficulties. Your doctor should be able to put you in touch with good advice about these aids and techniques, which ones are most suitable, how to obtain them, and financial or practical assistance if necessary.

With such a list of potential benefits it would be silly to let simple embarrassment or a reluctance to complain prevent you from obtaining medical advice, but are there any more substantial disadvantages to consulting your doctor? The main risk is to your morale. A family doctor has to recognize disorders in every system of the body so it is not reasonable to expect him to be expert on all of them; that is the job of specialist doctors. Not all doctors have heard of bladder training or pelvic floor exercise, the two main planks of the self-help program, and not all those who have heard of them believe that they are effective. (In Chapters 7 and 8 I give some of the scientific evidence for how well they do work, but you may find the word of one doctor face to face more convincing than any number of careful researchers reported at second hand.) It is very damaging if your doctor convinces you that the self-help scheme is likely to fail, because that robs you of the motivation to carry out the program properly and so makes it very difficult to achieve success.

If your particular doctor does not favour the use of bladder training or pelvic floor exercise he may say that there is no treatment suitable for your problem; this is immensely demoralizing. Alternatively he may encourage you to try some other treatment — drugs, perhaps, or surgery. There are occasions when these are appropriate but, as they always carry the risk of side effects, it is usually sensible to try the gentler treatments described in this book first. This is especially true of surgery where a first operation has a much better chance of success than any subsequent one so it is very important not to waste that first chance on an unnecessary or inappropriate operation. You do not have to accept any treatment you do not want, of course, but you may find it difficult and disagreeable to refuse.

In the end you will have to decide for yourself, knowing your own symptoms and your own doctor, whether you want to ask his advice. If you have mild or long-standing symptoms, or stress incontinence in the first few months after having a baby, it is perfectly reasonable to have a good try at beating the problem yourself before asking for extra help if you still need it. On the other hand, you should consult a doctor if any of the following apply:

1. if you have blood in your urine

2. if it is painful when you empty your bladder

3. if you feel that you need to empty your bladder again when you have only just finished emptying it once

4. if you have difficulty in starting to urinate, or a slow stream of urine when you do get started

5. if you have continuous dribbling incontinence

6. if you have other symptoms, even though they may not seem to be related to your bladder problem

7. if your problem came on suddenly after a long period of good bladder control (except stress incontinence after childbirth)

8. if your problem is making you very worried or very depressed

If you have symptoms 2 and/or 3 only, check whether they fit the description for cystitis in Chapter 11. If so, you can try a self-help treatment for a couple of days but you should see a doctor if the problem persists or recurs. I have already mentioned that it is particularly sensible to see a doctor if your symptoms seem to be related to the menopause, medicines or surgery.

# Getting Medical Help

The first thing to say here is that your doctor is not the only source of medical help, although he is usually the most appropriate person to see.

If you find the doctor very intimidating, you might find the clinic nurse or a health visitor more approachable in the first instance.

If your problem began in connection with childbirth, a maternity physiotherapist should be able to give good advice. You can make contact through the hospital where you had your baby, or talk to your community midwife.

In some areas there is a nurse with special responsibility for problems of continence; she usually has a title like 'continence adviser' and is attached to one of the larger hospitals where you may be able to contact her by phone. As she is a specialist dealing with bladder problems all the time you can be sure that she will not be disconcerted or dismissive however unusual your problem may seem to you. Consider the more usual sources of help first, though, as continence advisers are rather thin on the ground and would be overwhelmed with work if everyone with a bladder problem went straight to them.

There is no guarantee that, because a doctor is of a particular sex or a particular age, he or she will be more or less sympathetic or interested in your difficulties. All the same, doctors recognize that many women feel more comfortable with a woman doctor when they have very personal matters to discuss. If your doctor works as part of a group, it should not be difficult to arrange to see another member of the practice. Receptionists are generally very sensible and sensitive about this and do not even ask why but, if you do come across a more inquisitorial guardian of the appointments book, remember that you do not have to answer any personal questions she may ask. Just repeat firmly that you would particularly like to discuss the problem with a woman doctor. Emphasis on 'woman' is usually enough to get the point through. 'It's a personal matter; I'd rather not discuss it here' is a polite but effective block if you are asked any further unwelcome questions.

Naturally you want to choose the doctor who will be most understanding of your difficulties, but unless you know the doctors in the practice very well it will be difficult to guess who that will be. Unless you have a strong preference to see someone else, it is most sensible to see whichever doctor you have seen most often before. He knows you best and has the best chance of seeing the whole picture of your health rather than isolated symptoms.

Before you go to see the doctor it is worth preparing yourself so that you can get the best use out of a short appointment.

First of all, there is no need to feel apologetic for seeking medical advice. You should not expect to put up with incontinence at any age, you are not complaining unnecessarily and you are not wasting the doctor's time. Nor are you being lazy and looking for a magic cure. Seeing a doctor is one sensible step in trying to overcome your problem.

Secondly, there is no need to be afraid of what will happen at the appointment. The doctor will ask lots of questions and he may want a urine sample (which you would produce in private). He may not need to do a vaginal examination but if one is necessary and you hate the idea, do let him know. It is entirely routine from his point of view but he should understand your feelings if you find it thoroughly disagreeable.

Thirdly, try and talk yourself out of feeling embarrassed. This is partly a question of reminding yourself that the bladder is only a part of the body, not much different from a stomach or an ear, and partly it is a question of choosing what words to use. You will not shock your doctor however blunt you are so it is fine to use plain language (e.g. 'pee') if you feel most comfortable with it. On the other hand, he will be equally at home with formal medical terms (such as 'urinate') if you are happy using those. If you do not give a lead he may well use some euphemism such as 'pass water', not because that is necessarily the way he likes to talk but because he cannot tell whether you will understand the formal or be offended by the earthy.

The easiest way to introduce the subject is simply to say 'I've got a bladder problem' and then let the doctor take the initiative in asking questions to find out exactly what the problem is. Alternatively, you might say something like 'I can't cough without wetting myself' or 'I think I've got stress incontinence'. Make sure that he knows if there are any other factors which could be important such as the menopause, medicines taken for other illnesses, or major emotional upheavals like a divorce or a bereavement. Don't tell him that you have an unstable bladder or sphincter incompetence; you cannot be sure of that without elaborate tests and he will need to make his own diagnosis.

Think beforehand what it is you want your doctor to do for you. Half his patients will complain bitterly if they are not offered an instant cure while the other half will be furious if they are 'fobbed off' with a prescription. He has no way of telling which half you belong to unless you give him some clues! Let him know if all you want is advice or reassurance that there is no underlying disease.

If you are offered treatment or further investigations which you do not want, you do not have to take them. Neither do you have to be aggressive about refusing them. Explain that you would like to try to solve the problem with bladder training or pelvic floor exercise and ask whether you are going to come to any harm if you delay for three months or so before accepting any other treatment. Usually he will agree that there is no harm in it so you can go off home and get started. Let him know that you are glad of his advice and reassurance even though you are not taking up the offer of treatment at the moment, otherwise he will wonder why you bothered to consult him in the first place.

If the doctor seems dubious about your delaying three months before further action, you need to find out whether he is afraid that there may be a more serious problem or whether he is just dubious about self-help, so ask as many questions as you need to. If he has doubts about the value of the self-help treatment, find out whether they are general doubts or whether he thinks there is some particular reason why it would not be effective in your case. There is no point in arguing about whether your self-help program is going to work and it does not matter if he thinks you are a crank for wanting to try it. What does matter is that you get all the information you need to make your own decision. You do not want to reject effective or necessary treatment, but neither do you want to rush into anything irreversible.

# Chapter 4

# YOU, AND WHO ELSE?

Six weeks after the birth of my first baby, my doctor told me that I was only the second woman to complain of stress incontinence in the last three years of his experience. This was a doctor that I liked and trusted but there was never one moment when I believed that my situation could be so unusual. At the time, I had no evidence to back up my disbelief: it was simply unthinkable that, after keeping so fit through such a straightforward pregnancy and birth, I could have suffered an injury so rare as to appear only twice in three years. 'Only the second?' I mused sourly. 'Only the second to complain, maybe, but there must be an awful lot of young mothers out there keeping quiet!'

Later, when I studied the medical research literature, I discovered two things. First, I was right in guessing that the problem was really very widespread. Second, it is not only young mothers who are keeping quiet about their difficulties in bladder control. Incontinence is commoner amongst women than amongst men, commoner in women who have borne children and commoner in the elderly than in the young, but it is a substantial problem amongst people of all ages, all backgrounds and both sexes.

You do not need the information in this chapter in order to follow your treatment program but you may well be interested to see just how many people share your problem. It also casts a little light on some of the causes of bladder problems.

# Overall Prevalence of Incontinence

It is surprising that before 1980 no survey had been carried out to establish the prevalence of incontinence in the general population. The earlier studies involved selected groups of people, such as nurses, university students or patients attending hospitals for various reasons, and there is no guarantee that these groups show the same patterns of incontinence as people in general.

It is always difficult (and expensive) to carry out a survey on a representative population and on a large enough scale to give really meaningful results. In fact, it is more difficult than you might imagine even to interpret the responses to a questionnaire on this subject, not least because the subjects themselves give inconsistent answers. For example, in one study, a substantial number of women who answered 'Never' to the question 'Do you ever lose urine accidentally (against your wishes)?' then answered 'Yes' when asked 'Do you ever lose urine when bladder is full with sneezing or coughing?'.[4]

However, Thomas and co-workers completed an excellent large-scale survey of incontinence in the general population and published the results in 1980 and 1986.[30,31] They studied a real cross-section of the population by approaching all the people aged 5 and over on the lists of 12 family doctors in various parts of the UK — 22,430 of them. Some had moved but of the 20,398 who were still at the same address, 18,084 filled in and returned the questionnaire. As a check, the workers also interviewed 178 of the people who reported that they lost urine accidentally; they gave broadly the same answers during interview as on the questionnaires so the researchers could be fairly sure that the written replies were reliable. Incontinence was clearly defined ('involuntary excretion or leakage of urine in inappropriate places or at inappropriate times regardless of the quantity of urine lost') and if leaks occurred two or more times in a month, the incontinence was regarded as regular. Table 1 shows some of the results from this survey.

Regular incontinence affects women more than men at most ages. Nine per cent of all women aged 15 years old or more had regular

| Age Group | occasionally incontinent (less than twice a month) | | regularly incontinent (twice or more a month) | |
|---|---|---|---|---|
| | women (%) | men (%) | women (%) | men (%) |
| 5-14 | 11 | 11 | 5 | 7 |
| 15-34 | 16 | 2 | 5 | 1 |
| 35-64 | 20 | 4 | 11 | 2 |
| 65-84 | 14 | 9 | 11 | 7 |
| 85+ | 16 | 3 | 16 | 15 |

Table 1

incontinence compared to 2½ per cent of men aged 15 and over with the same difficulty. Up to the age of 14, both sexes appear to be affected equally. There is more bedwetting amongst the boys but this is roughly balanced by the urge incontinence more commonly found amongst the girls.

For the people with regular incontinence who were interviewed, the research team also assessed the severity of their symptoms. Between 20 and 30 per cent had moderate to severe incontinence which required extra laundry, pads and expenses and which restricted their activities. Roughly 50 per cent had minimal incontinence, with no restrictions, pads or expenses. The rest were considered to have slight incontinence although they had to wear pads occasionally and had some extra laundry. If those who were interviewed are representative, this means that of all women over the age of 15, approximately 2 per cent have regular moderate or severe incontinence, 3 per cent have regular slight incontinence and 4 per cent have regular minimal incontinence.

Yarnell[36] found a similar but slightly higher prevalence of incontinence by interviewing a thousand women in South Wales. 13 per cent of women aged 17 or more had episodes of incontinence at least once a week, and a further 31 per cent had very occasional leaks. 7 per cent considered that their bladder's behaviour constituted 'a problem', 3½ per cent felt that their social or domestic lives were restricted and 2½ per cent had daily or continuous wetting of their clothes.

The picture given by 800 women in Leicestershire is very much the same.[16] 41 per cent had incontinence of some degree, 6 per cent wore protection all the time and 15 per cent wore pads for exercise. Women in Denmark[27] and New Zealand[12] suffer in the same way with 30-40 per cent admitting to incontinence on occasions and 5-6 per cent troubled daily, often or always.

Both Yarnell and Thomas included questions in their surveys to try to identify the types of incontinence present. They found similar results. Of women with regular incontinence, 40 to 50 per cent had pure stress incontinence, 20 to 25 per cent had pure urge incontinence and about 30 per cent had mixed urge and stress incontinence. The proportions are similar for women with occasional incontinence.[27,12] Thomas also included a question about bedwetting but did not report the results for children over the age of 14. However, we can calculate that approximately 5 per cent of the regularly incontinent women had a problem other than simple or combined stress or urge incontinence.

Amongst patients arriving at a urological clinic, there is a smaller proportion (only 25 per cent) suffering from pure stress incontinence and a much larger proportion (20 per cent) with the less common problems of continuous incontinence or bedwetting.[7] This presumably reflects the fact that the latter difficulties are more distressing whereas simple stress incontinence is often a nuisance which can be lived with.

One report shows very clearly the extent to which women with incontinence do live with it rather than approaching a doctor for help in the early stages.[19] Almost 40 per cent of the incontinent patients arriving for treatment had had their symptoms for between two and ten years; 30 per cent had had them for longer than ten years! At another clinic, half the patients had had their symptoms for four years or longer by the time they came for treatment.[34] In Yarnell's study, too, as in Holst's and others, it is striking how few women sought medical help. Certainly many had mild incontinence which they considered to be a minor nuisance rather than a medical problem, but even amongst the women who felt that their incontinence was restricting their lives, only half had sought help.

# Prevalence of Particular Symptoms

## Stress Incontinence

From the large-scale surveys described already we can estimate that between 6 and 10 per cent of adult women have regular stress incontinence with leaks occurring more than twice a month. About three-fifths of these have pure stress incontinence while the remaining two-fifths have stress and urge incontinence combined. These surveys found that a further 20 to 30 per cent of women had occasional incontinence, roughly three-quarters of it either stress incontinence or combined stress and urge incontinence. Presumably the earlier studies[6,22,35] of young nurses and students which found very large numbers (50 to 65 per cent) of them suffering from urine leakage on coughing, sneezing or laughing included women whose mishaps occurred very seldom, although a proportion (2 to 16 per cent) were reported as having urinary accidents frequently.

## Urgency and Urge Incontinence

According to the major surveys, 2 to 3 per cent of adult women suffer regularly from urge incontinence without associated stress incontinence. There is less information about the proportion of women who, while never actually leaking, have to rush to reach the toilet although Bungay[3] claimed that 15 to 20 per cent of women between the ages of 30 and 60 had this symptom of urinary urgency. Sommer's study[27] suggests a figure nearer 25 per cent as 40 per cent of the women in it had urgency but only 13 per cent had actual urge incontinence.

## Frequency and Nocturia

Sommer found these symptoms to be very widespread. Over half the women emptied their bladders more often than 3-hourly during the day and 11 per cent were visiting the toilet more often than 2-hourly. 14 per cent were getting up twice or more in the night and about a third of these were disturbed at least three times each night.

Nocturia becomes commoner with increasing age and studies restricted to younger women show smaller proportions affected.[10,28]

## Bedwetting

Bedwetting has been carefully studied in young people. Two large surveys[5,24] agree that the prevalence is close to 1½ per cent for girls and 3 per cent for boys in their mid-teens but no study has reported the prevalence of bedwetting in a representative sample of adults. Such reports as there are concern men recruited into the American army or navy and these suggest that at the age of 20 about 1 per cent of these young men wet the bed.[18,32] It is not clear whether adult women are more or less susceptible to bedwetting than adult men; some clinics find a preponderance of men amongst their patients while others find an even distribution.

## Giggle Incontinence

Common experience tells us that many adults encounter urinary urgency when they laugh (how else could the phrase 'I nearly wet myself' have become so widespread?), and many children actually wet their pants if the event is funny enough. There is a spectrum of responses to laughter and there are more people than you might guess at the end of the spectrum where laughter provokes actual urine leakage.

Glahn's study[9] seems to be the only one which aimed to find out about the prevalence of giggle incontinence specifically. Of 99 student nurses aged 19 to 26 years, nine felt an acute need to reach a toilet during laughter and six of these actually suffered urine leakage. A further fifteen remembered suffering from leakage or urgency with laughter when they were younger.

In earlier reports, before the term giggle micturition was invented, anyone losing urine on laughter was considered to have stress incontinence. For example, Nemir and Middleton[22] found that 26 per cent of the young women entering the first year of university in the early 1950s suffered from 'stress incontinence', at least occasionally, when laughing or excited but not when coughing or sneezing. This is not the usual pattern of urine loss with stress incontinence and today we might guess that some of these women had giggle incontinence.

## Incontinence During Intercourse

Incontinence during sexual activity is not unusual but women who experience it are likely to be so embarrassed that they will not mention it to their doctor even if they pluck up the courage to discuss their other episodes of stress or urge incontinence. Hilton[11] found that about a quarter of the women referred to the gynaecological urology clinic suffered from urine leakage during intercourse, but only two out of 79 volunteered this information before they were asked directly. The proportion is similar for those with genuine stress incontinence and for those with bladder instability but the details are different. You are more likely to leak on penetration if you have stress incontinence and more likely to leak at orgasm if you have an unstable bladder.

## Cystitis

Cystitis is episodic with each attack only lasting for a few days so at any particular time the number of women affected is fairly small, but over a year or two a very large number of women will suffer one or more attacks. Iosif found that 40 per cent of Swedish women between 21 and 70 years old had received treatment for urinary tract infection in the previous two years.[15] Rees found that a similar proportion of the women attending a family planning clinic had a history of definite cystitis and that a further 20 per cent had had symptoms of possible cystitis.[23]

Some women never have cystitis and a few have a single isolated bout but, in general, if you have an attack of cystitis you should take it as a warning that, unless you take a few precautions, you will be prone to further attacks in the future. Over half of the women who are treated for one urinary tract infection have another attack within two years and if you have had repeated urinary tract infections (three or more), you have a 50 per cent chance of recurrence within five months.[20]

# The Effect of Ageing and the Menopause

The table on page 27 shows how incontinence becomes more prevalent with increasing age. In women, the increase is apparent from early middle age while in men the prevalence of incontinence does not rise markedly until retirement age. The increased prevalence of incontinence in women in their twenties and thirties is largely due to the effect of childbearing but there is also a direct effect of ageing which becomes more marked as the years roll on.

The prevalence of combined stress and urge incontinence increases with age and is the commonest form of incontinence in women over the age of 75. Pure stress incontinence becomes more widespread up to the age of 55 and is the commonest form of incontinence throughout middle life. In later years, the prevalence of pure stress incontinence falls while pure urge and combined incontinence increase in importance. The reduced prevalence of stress incontinence in older women has been noted in other studies;[2,36,12] there is no clear explanation for it although we may guess that as their muscular strength diminishes, women are less able to subject their bladders to the sudden stresses which previously produced leaks.

In older women incontinence increases not only in prevalence but also in severity. Although most women with regular incontinence are affected only minimally or slightly at all ages, the proportion affected so severely as to need help from others rises from 3 per cent in those under 65 to 15 per cent in women above this age.

The influence of the menopause is not so clear. A substantial proportion of women with incontinence date the start of their difficulty to their menopause. For example, Beck and Hsu[1] found that 60 out of 95 postmenopausal women had a degree of incontinence; 32 of them said that it had begun at the menopause and a further 14 said that existing symptoms had worsened then. Iosif[15] questioned 512 women between the ages of 20 and 70 who suffered from stress incontinence and found that a third of them too had first developed their symptoms after the menopause.

On the other hand, a study of 515 45-year-old women in Denmark[13] found no difference in the prevalence of incontinence between those who had passed the menopause and those who had not, and Jolleys[16] actually found the prevalence lower in women after the menopause (35 per cent) than before (48 per cent).

# The Effect of Pregnancy and Childbirth

Urinary symptoms are so common as to be customary during pregnancy and generally become more severe as the pregnancy progresses. Frequent urination is regarded as a classic symptom of early pregnancy; it affects about half of all pregnant women within the first three months and the vast majority (75 to 95 per cent) find themselves urinating seven or more times a day towards the end of the pregnancy. Night-time urination is not quite so common but still affects about a quarter of pregnant women in the early months and up to three-quarters towards term.[28]

These effects are not permanent and after the birth the pattern of urination soon returns to normal so that frequency and nocturia are no more usual in women who have had children than in those who have not.

Incontinence during pregnancy is also very prevalent. Unlike frequency and nocturia which are more of a problem in first pregnancies, incontinence tends to occur more commonly in second and subsequent pregnancies. Urge incontinence affects 10 to 20 per cent of women near the end of pregnancy and stress incontinence has been variously estimated as affecting anywhere between 30 and 85 per cent of pregnant women at some stage.[8,28,33]

In some cases, the birth itself may produce damage which causes stress incontinence and between 10 and 20 per cent of women with stress incontinence attribute it to the birth of one of their children. In general, though, the incontinence which is experienced during pregnancy becomes less severe soon after the birth and may even disappear completely. However, a number of women never completely recover their bladder control and continue to experience accidental urine loss.

Francis studied 400 pregnant women in 1960[8] and found that about a third of them never suffered from incontinence either during the pregnancy or afterwards. A further third had stress incontinence during the pregnancy which cleared up completely soon after delivery. Most of the remainder had stress incontinence during pregnancy and on occasions afterwards, generally when they had a cough; about one in twenty had severe stress incontinence permanently after the birth.

Iosif[14] questioned 1411 mothers shortly after their babies were born and found a rather smaller proportion (about a quarter) of them with stress incontinence. Three quarters of these women said that their incontinence had begun during pregnancy and a fifth that it had started following the birth. Just over half of them found that their incontinence resolved itself within three months, leaving about 10 per cent with a permanent problem.

The major survey by Thomas and associates agreed that about 10 per cent of women with one, two or three children have incontinence on a regular basis, and found that the problem affects an even larger proportion (16 per cent) of women with four or more children. Regular incontinence is much less prevalent amongst women with no children, only 3 to 4 per cent of whom are affected.

Other studies suggest that the problem is actually more widespread. Sommer[27] found stress incontinence in 32 per cent of women with children compared to 12 per cent of those without. In one general practice in Britain[16] roughly half of the women with children had incontinence (slightly less of those with one or two children and slightly more of those with three or four); it was three times less common in the women without children. In the second study,[25,26] researchers managed to recontact 643 out of a thousand mothers who had given birth three years earlier. About a third of them still had stress incontinence to some extent; 10 per cent wore pads sometimes and over 10 per cent had leaks more often than once a week.

The original focus of the second study mentioned above had been episiotomy. There were a thousand mothers helping in the study, split into two groups. In one group, the midwives used episiotomy liberally to prevent tears; in the other, they used it sparingly, only performing an episiotomy if the baby was getting into difficulties. In the 'liberal' group, half of the mothers ended up having an episiotomy, and in the 'sparing' group only a tenth, but it made no difference to their chances of having incontinence three months or three years later.

Other workers[14,33] agree that the occurrence of an episiotomy or a tear during birth has little effect on the likelihood of the mother having incontinence afterwards. They also find that the weight of the baby, the whole length of the labour and the length of the second stage of labour have no measurable effect on the prevalence of postnatal incontinence. At first sight this is surprising as you might well expect the birth of a large baby to cause more injury than a smaller one, and a very long or a very fast labour to have more damaging consequences for the muscles of the pelvic floor. The whole process of childbearing undoubtedly puts a woman's continence mechanism at risk but it seems to be the pregnancy which is the most significant factor, the details of the birth being relatively unimportant.

# Chapter 5

# HOW THE URINARY SYSTEM WORKS – OR DOESN'T

If you are keen to start your self-help program immediately, you can skip this chapter for now and go straight on to Chapter 6. However, you will find it worthwhile to come back and read it later as it will help you to understand what has probably gone wrong and how the treatments are supposed to work.

## The Urinary System

Urine is produced in the two kidneys. Production can be speeded up if the body needs to offload excess water or slowed down to conserve water, but it can never be switched off completely. As soon as it is formed, the urine flows away from the kidney down a tube which enters the bladder near its base. There is a valve on each tube at the point where it enters the bladder so that in normal health urine never flows back up to the kidneys. The kidneys and the tubes connecting them to the bladder form the upper urinary tract which is beyond the scope of this book.

The bladder is made of extremely stretchy muscle so that it can expand to accommodate the constantly arriving urine without the pressure inside rising very much. At an appropriate time, the muscle contracts and squirts the urine out through the urethra.

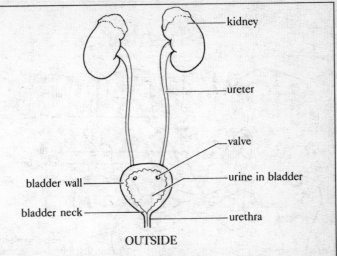

kidney

ureter

valve

bladder wall

urine in bladder

bladder neck

urethra

OUTSIDE

**Figure 1:** Schematic diagram of the urinary system seen from the front.

The muscle of the bladder wall is called the detrusor muscle. The walls of the urethra are also muscular.

The kidneys are packed in fat and firmly attached to the back, in the abdominal cavity, each slightly to one side of the spine.

The urethra is a tube which leads from the neck of the bladder to the outside of the body. It has a soft inner layer which helps to form a leakproof seal when the sides of the tube are pressed together. There are muscles in and around the wall of the urethra which contract to squeeze it shut and relax to allow for urine flow.

The bones of the pelvis form a ring, rather like a bowl with a hole in the bottom (Figure 2). The bladder lies in the front part of this bowl with the uterus behind it and the rectum behind that. Above these are the other abdominal organs, including the large bulk of the intestines. The bones are curved in a way which gives some support to the internal organs but the main support from below is given by a set of muscles which largely fill in the hole in the 'bowl' and form a floor to the pelvis.

There are several different muscles in a complicated arrangement

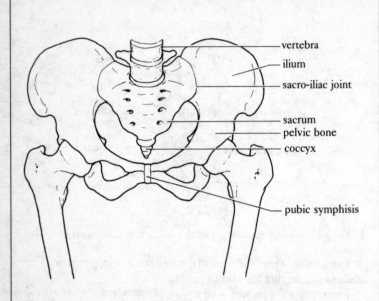

**Figure 2:** Sketch of the bones of the pelvis seen from the front.

The sacrum is a solid bone formed from several vertebrae; the lowest part of it is called the coccyx or tailbone. The pelvic bones form a pair firmly joined together at the pubic symphysis in front, and attached to the sacrum through the sacro-iliac joints at the back. There is normally little movement at these joints, especially the pubic symphysis, but they become slightly more mobile and vulnerable to injury during pregnancy when the ligaments soften. Pain in the sacro-iliac joints (low in the back, off-centre) is common in both men and women.

The 'wing' part of the pelvic bone which sweeps up to form the point of the hip is called the ilium, and the ischium is the part which extends downwards to take your weight in the sitting position. The front part of the two pelvic bones together forms the pubic bone.

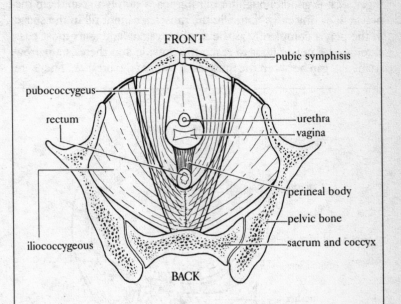

**Figure 3:** Schematic diagram of the major pelvic floor muscles seen from above.

The most important of the pelvic floor muscles for urinary control is the pubococcygeus which runs from the pubic bone backwards. Some of its fibres connect to the perineal body between the anus and the vagina, and some connect to the walls of the anal canal, but the main attachments are behind the anus to the coccyx and to the muscle of the other side. The iliococcygeus is a thinner muscle connecting the ilium of the pelvic bone to the coccyx or to the muscle of the opposite side. The ischiococcygeus, not shown on this diagram, connects the ischium of the pelvic bone to the coccyx.

These muscles together form the levator ani (i.e. anus-lifting) muscles.

The urethra is linked to the pelvic bones by ligaments running diagonally forward which should prevent it moving any great distance backwards.

(even Figure 3 is very much simplified) but since they all work together it is good enough for our purposes simply to call them the pelvic floor muscles. Naturally the muscles cannot fill in the space in the pelvis completely as the urethra, vagina and anus must pass through the pelvic floor to reach the outside and there is a narrow triangular gap between the muscles in front of the urethra. There are

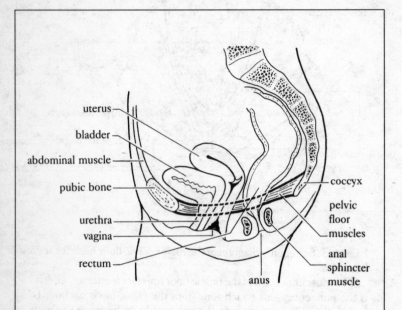

**Figure 4:** Schematic diagram of the pelvis, its contents, and the pelvic floor muscles seen from the left side.

The urethra is closely connected to the front wall of the vagina. It is also attached to the pubic bone and the front part of the pelvic floor muscles by a band of tissue containing ligament and muscle.

The uterus is remarkably small when non-pregnant and cannot be felt above the pubic bone, but it does have very thick muscular walls to allow it to stretch enough to hold a full-grown baby.

There is a ring of muscle around the anus, the anal sphincter, below the pelvic floor muscles.

other muscles below the pelvic floor muscles, nearer the skin, but these are less important in the support of the pelvic organs.

Figure 4 shows the main pelvic organs in side view and Figure 5 is an external view of the perineum. It is well worth propping yourself up on a couple of pillows and having a look at your perineum with a mirror. You may be surprised to find how close your urethra is to

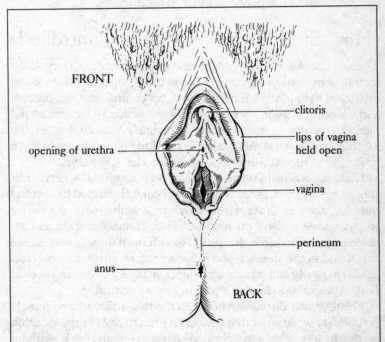

**Figure 5:** Sketch to show the main features of the perineum, seen from between the legs of a person lying on her back.

The appearance of the perineal area varies a great deal from one person to another so yours may look quite different from this. It depends partly on whether you have had children but is also largely a matter of inbuilt individual difference. 'Perineum' is often used to indicate the whole of the area between the legs (the saddle area) but doctors and midwives usually use it to refer to the area between the vagina and the anus.

your vagina, for example, as the sensation of urine flowing over your clitoris can give the impression that the urethra opens there. You will also be able to see whether the walls of your vagina bulge towards the entrance, and (without the mirror) you may be able to feel your pelvic floor muscles. They press against the sides of the vagina about half a finger's length inside. There is more detail on how to check the condition of the pelvic muscles in Chapter 7.

# How the Urinary System is Controlled

The amount of urine you produce, and its concentration, is regulated by way of hormones which circulate in the blood and influence the activity of the kidneys. You have no direct control over this process and it is only occasionally a factor in incontinence. In most cases the difficulty is not in the quantity of urine produced but in the mechanisms which should keep it in the bladder until an appropriate time. These mechanisms depend on muscles and nerves.

There are two main types of muscle, both governed by nerves but subject to varying degrees of intentional control. Striped (voluntary) muscles, such as those which move your limbs, have distinctive stripes visible under a microscope. They contract quickly and are responsive to conscious decision. Smooth (involuntary) muscle like that found in the stomach and intestine has no stripes; it contracts relatively slowly and you have no direct voluntary command over it. Both types of muscle play a part in urinary control.

The textbook distinction between the two is that striped muscle is voluntary while smooth is involuntary but in real life the situation is much less clear-cut. Striped muscles often work without conscious effort and in practice smooth muscles can be influenced, though not directly, from the thinking level of the brain.

For an example of the various ways in which a striped muscle can be controlled, think of the leg muscles. If you decide to bend your knee, a signal goes from your brain through nerves in the spinal cord and then along a peripheral nerve to the appropriate muscle in your leg which promptly contracts and bends the knee; this is a classical voluntary movement. However, lower centres in the brain can organize the repetitive movements needed for an activity like walking without your having to think about it, and nerve pathways in the spine are quite enough to produce a reflex contraction of appropriate muscles and jerk your foot away if you tread on something sharp. The striped muscles relevant to urinary control are governed on a similar variety of levels.

A good example of smooth muscle would be the stomach. Most of the time it carries out its regular churning movements using only local nerve networks for coordination but it still has connections with the central nervous system. If you eat bad food, for instance, a centre in the brain can coordinate the contractions of various muscles (including the smooth muscles of the stomach) which result in the ejection of the offending meal from the body. You have little conscious control over this process, though you may be able to delay it for a short time rather as you can delay emptying a very full bladder for a short time.

You cannot directly signal smooth muscle to contract but you have two indirect ways of exerting influence. One way is by thinking; in the same way that you can affect your heartbeat by thinking peaceful or stirring thoughts, you can influence your stomach with greedy or gruesome ones. The other way is by using your voluntary muscles to set off reflexes involving the involuntary ones, for example moving your fingers to tickle the back of your throat with obvious unpleasant consequences. For an adult, control over the smooth muscle of the urinary system is so habitual that it is often not conscious but it surely works in the same ways.

All types of muscle are susceptible to emotional influences. Many of these reactions seem quite pointless but they are still not easily controlled. Many people blush when embarrassed (a reaction of smooth muscle in blood vessels) and most of us find our skeletal muscles shivering intensely if we have been badly frightened, even when we are uninjured. The urinary system is not exempt from such effects so nervousness, for example, may well encourage the bladder muscle to contract.

The muscles of the bladder, urethra and pelvic floor all have nerve connections with the spinal cord which can organize reflex actions. There are further connections via the spinal cord to various levels of the brain. It is these pathways which allow conscious awareness of the bladder and related muscles and permit influence by deliberate decision and by emotion.

To store and void urine effectively requires the close coordination of several muscles. During storage, the urethral muscles contract to keep the outlet tube closed while the muscle of the bladder should remain relaxed so that the pressure inside does not increase greatly as it fills. During urination, the pelvic floor and urethral muscles relax to reduce the resistance to urine flow and the detrusor contracts so that the urine is actively expelled.

The bladder contains sensors which signal the degree of fullness by detecting the degree of stretch (not pressure) in the bladder wall. There is a centre in the spinal cord which, receiving the message from the sensors that the bladder is full, can organize the muscle activities to empty it completely. This is a reflex action; it does not need input from the brain and it is presumably how the bladder empties in babies and in people with spinal injuries where messages cannot pass between the lower spinal centres and the brain.

The detrusor (bladder muscle) is a smooth muscle so deliberate influence over it works indirectly. In a healthy adult, signals from the brain inhibit the spinal reflex emptying of the bladder. Voiding does not occur either until this inhibition is consciously lifted or until the stretch in the bladder wall makes the sensors signal so furiously that the inhibition is overridden (in the same way that you would eventually be forced by reflex to breathe no matter how hard you tried to hold your breath).

Information from the stretch sensors is transmitted to conscious levels of the brain where it is interpreted (rather unreliably) as a sensation of bladder fullness or need to urinate. A person with strong bladder control can then choose to delay urinating until much later or at least for long enough to find a suitable place to empty her bladder conveniently. Once there, without even having to think about it, she can release the inhibition of voiding and allow the spinal reflexes to take over.

The detrusor muscle is normally quite capable of emptying the bladder without help from the abdominal muscles but quite a number of people use abdominal pressure to start the stream off. It may be that by pressing with the abdominal muscles while relaxing the pelvic floor they can stretch the bladder wall near the bladder neck and trigger the stretch sensors to set off the emptying reflex.

No doubt the process of urination is helped by the regular association between the toilet and bladder emptying just as, if you have a regular eating place, your body thoughtlessly prepares itself for food on the way there. Even imagining a toilet can make matters worse if you are already having difficulty in holding on after feeling an urge to void.

To hold urine securely in the bladder, the detrusor muscle should stay relaxed and the muscles in and around the urethra should contract to hold the outlet shut. It is not quite clear how much direct voluntary control we have over the muscles in the urethra (there has been some disagreement over whether there is striped as well as smooth muscle in its wall and whether it is served by the usual sort of nerves) but if you can stop the flow of urine quickly in midstream, you must be contracting muscles in or very close to the wall of the urethra at will. Contracting the pelvic floor muscles also tends to reduce urine flow but pelvic floor contraction alone is not enough to close the urethra as the muscles do not completely surround it.

Most men have very good control of their urinary streams and can shut them off completely in less than a second without having had any previous practice. Some women can do the same, so the necessary muscles and nerves must be present in both sexes. However, many perfectly healthy women cannot stop their stream so quickly and quite a number cannot stop it at all. Duncan[1] questioned 134 women, mostly young and having had no children, and found that over a third of them were wholly or partially unable to interrupt urination. They lacked either the required strength in the muscles or the coordination in the nerves, but perhaps they could learn the coordination and build up the strength with practice. If the stream can be interrupted only after a delay of five to fifteen seconds, this indicates that voluntary muscle is not being used; instead there is inhibition of the bladder contraction followed by passive closure of the bladder neck.

The pelvic floor muscles are certainly striped muscles and should be accessible to voluntary control but, like the muscles which wiggle your ears, not everyone is aware of them and not everyone has learned to work them consciously. However, it is said that, with the aid of a small mirror and a large amount of patience, anyone can learn to wiggle their ears so you can expect that, no matter how recalcitrant your pelvic floor muscles may seem to be at the moment, you will eventually gain conscious control over them.

Striped muscles come in two sorts. 'Fast twitch' muscle contracts very quickly but it soon becomes fatigued and cannot hold a contraction for long periods. 'Slow twitch' muscle contracts more slowly (though not so slowly as smooth muscle) but it is resistant to fatigue. The pelvic floor muscles are of mixed type. Most of the fibres are slow and are presumably responsible for the tone of the muscle, i.e. the background tension which normally prevails apart from particular episodes of relaxation or contraction. There are also some fast twitch fibres which allow for a speedy response in reflex or voluntary activity.

# Continence During Physical Activity and the Role of the Pelvic Floor

Practically any physical activity causes the pressure in the abdomen to rise as the abdominal muscles tense to support and stabilize the body. Simply moving from a lying to a sitting position increases abdominal pressure, and running, jumping or lifting heavy weights naturally increase it more. Coughing and sneezing involve sharp, short-lived increases in pressure as the muscles contract suddenly to push air forcefully out of the lungs.

As the bladder lies in the abdomen, any increase in abdominal pressure tends to compress it and squeeze urine out. However, two factors counteract this tendency and help to maintain continence. The first (and probably more important) factor is completely passive, depending on the fact that the upper part of the urethra lies above the pelvic floor in the abdomen as shown in Figure 6a. With the bladder neck and upper urethra closed, and supported by a firm pelvic floor, the same pressure rise which tends to compress the bladder compresses the urethra equally. The forces acting to eject urine are matched by forces acting to retain it, and no additional muscular activity is needed to prevent a leak.

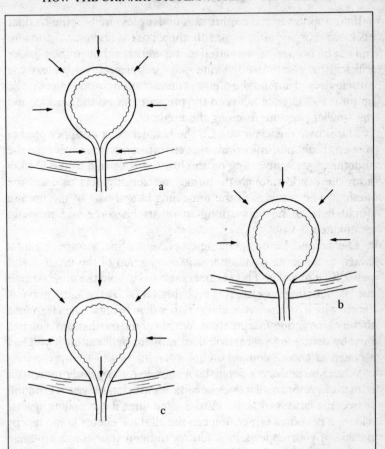

**Figure 6:** Schematic view of the bladder, upper urethra and pelvic floor muscles to show the effect of raised pressure in the abdomen.

6a Bladder and urethra well supported above a firm pelvic floor. Abdominal pressure acts on the upper urethra (keeping it closed) as well as on the bladder.

6b Weakened support. Abdominal pressure does not reach the urethra.

6c Open bladder neck. Abdominal pressure reaches the urethra through the urine and tends to open it.

If the support of the urethra sags under pressure or if the bladder neck has dropped as in Figure 6b, then a rise in abdominal pressure will not be properly transmitted to the urethra although the bladder will still be compressed. Urine will be squeezed out unless the muscles in and around the urethra contract strongly enough to make up for the difference between the pressure put on the bladder and the smaller pressure reaching the urethra.

The situation is even worse if the bladder neck or upper urethra is open. Fluid transmits pressure very efficiently so in this case the abdominal pressure acting on the bladder is carried to the urethra from the inside through the urine and actually acts to open the urethra. The muscles of the remaining closed part of the urethra would have to be very strong to resist this force and maintain continence.

The second factor operating to prevent urine leakage during a cough or a sneeze is an automatic contraction of the urethral and pelvic floor muscles. This contraction helps to hold the urine despite the sudden pressure rise. It is probably set off by the same nervous centre which organizes the cough rather than being a reflex response to the rising abdominal pressure. Whatever the mechanism, you can help by tightening your pelvic floor muscles deliberately if you feel a cough or sneeze coming on.

When you activate a pelvic floor muscle (or any other muscle) it tries to shorten, and if it does become shorter lengthwise it is bound to become fatter widthwise. At the same time, if it is pulling against a load, it becomes firmer. You can see all three effects in the biceps muscle of your upper arm if you try to bend your elbow up while holding something heavy.

The pelvic muscles are slung like a pair of hammocks between the pubic bone and the tailbone. The only way the muscles can shorten when you tighten them is by lifting to lie in a straighter line. Figure 7 shows this in an exaggerated way. The effect of this lifting and tightening is to make a more definite floor to the pelvis (more like a tightly stretched trampoline than a sagging hammock) so that abdominal pressure is transmitted more effectively to the parts of the urethra lying above it.

As the muscles shorten they must also fatten which has the effect

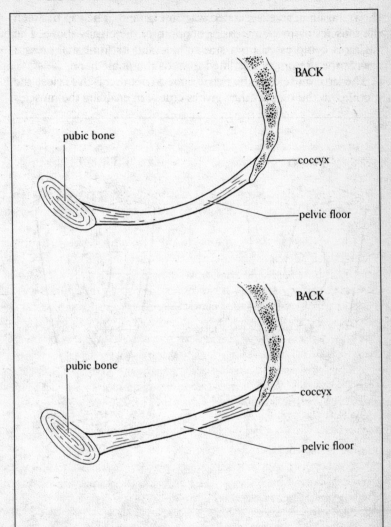

**Figure 7:** An exaggerated view of the movement of the pelvic floor muscles seen from the side.
7a Muscles relaxed ('hammock')
7b Muscles contracted ('trampoline')

shown, again in an exaggerated way, in Figure 8. The gap between the muscles narrows, increasing support for the organs above. The vagina is compressed from side to side and its front wall presses against the urethra as it is lifted towards the pubic bone.

The large muscles of the pelvic floor do not themselves close the urethra but the support they give is crucial in enabling the muscles

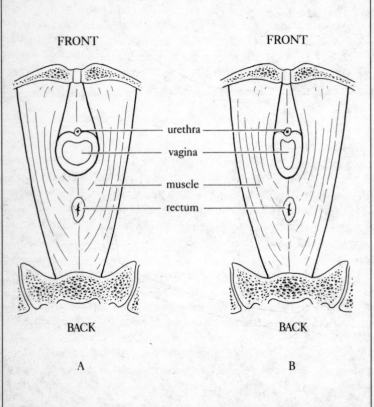

**Figure 8:** An exaggerated view of the movement of the pelvic floor seen from above.
  8a Muscles relaxed
  8b Muscles contracted

of the urethra and bladder neck to prevent urine loss during physical stress.

# What Goes Wrong and How

'Bladder problem' is handy shorthand to cover almost any symptom involving urine or urination but very often the source of the difficulty is not in the bladder itself. The system for producing, storing and voiding urine to suit both bodily need and social convenience has many components, any one of which can malfunction. We can think of four separate areas which may cause problems: urine production, the lower urinary tract itself (i.e. the bladder and urethra), the supporting structures and the coordinating system.

## Disorders of Urine Production

Urine carries waste products and water out of the body so its production must be closely controlled to remove the right amounts of each. A problem in this department needs medical treatment, and if the problem is that the kidneys cannot produce urine fast enough to remove waste efficiently, it needs urgent treatment. The person might not notice any urinary symptoms but would feel ill in other ways. Overproduction of urine is less serious in itself but still needs treatment.

People with untreated diabetes insipidus produce vast volumes of very dilute urine because they do not have enough of a hormone called vasopressin (anti-diuretic hormone) which normally allows the kidneys to take excess water back from the urine into the bloodstream. They must empty their bladders frequently day and night but apart from a few (presumably heavy sleepers) who develop bedwetting they are not generally incontinent. Untreated diabetes mellitus (ordinary sugar diabetes) also causes excessive urine production with similar consequences.

Normally the body produces extra vasopressin at night which slows overnight urine production. Failure to do so might contribute to nocturia or bedwetting.

# Disorders Within the Bladder or Urethra

Faults in the gross structure of the bladder or urethra are uncommon causes of urinary problems. There can be abnormal connections from the upper urethra, the bladder or even the upper urinary tract to the outside which cause continuous dribbling of urine; these may be inborn or the result of injury, but they are rare. Sometimes the bladder develops pouches from which the urine does not empty completely and these make bladder infections much more probable.

Partial blockage of the urethra is unusual in women but widespread in older men. It leads to a slow stream of urine, seldom itself a major nuisance, but the more annoying symptoms of frequency, urgency and nocturia generally follow. These should not be ignored as it is important for the obstruction to be cleared.

Inflammation of the bladder or urethra, owing to infection or whatever else, is likely to make them oversensitive and give rise to urgency or even urge incontinence. Frequency of urination follows from the sensation of urgency, and urinating from an inflamed bladder or through an inflamed urethra is generally painful. These are the symptoms of cystitis.

The bladder neck and urethra need to be pliant in order to close effectively. Scar tissue is relatively stiff so scarring as a result of injury or surgery weakens the seal and predisposes to incontinence.

As well as having flexible walls, the urethra has a resilient lining which acts to make a leakproof seal by squashing into all the little crevices like the thin foam strip of draught excluder around a window frame. The cells of this lining, like those lining the vagina, are sensitive to sex hormones, particularly oestrogen. As the levels of hormones fluctuate, the urethral lining waxes and wanes in response. It becomes thinner before a period, after a baby and, most especially, after the menopause, so stress incontinence is more likely at these times. Urgency may be a problem too as the thinner lining is more easily irritated. Oral contraceptives mimic sex hormones so they too may affect bladder control in sensitive people.

# Disorders of Support

Weakness in the muscles and ligaments supporting the urethra and bladder neck is more of a factor in stress incontinence than in any of the other bladder problems. Muscle weakness may be caused by direct damage to muscles but it can also be caused indirectly by injury to nerves. In women with stress incontinence, there is clear evidence of damage to the nerves supplying the urethral and pelvic floor muscle[5,6] as well as damage to the pelvic floor muscle itself[2].

Most of the women who consult a doctor about stress incontinence have had at least one child, and in many of them the incontinence dates back to when they had the baby, so it is an obvious suggestion that the supporting structures are damaged during childbirth. Clearly the pelvic floor muscles are severely stretched in the course of a vaginal birth, just as the abdominal muscles are stretched in the course of a pregnancy, and are very lax in the immediate aftermath. There is also a good chance of some injury to the nerves supplying the pelvic floor and urethra.

However, most of this damage is reversible and there is less permanent ill effect than you might think from looking at the tissues immediately after the birth. Stretched muscle regains its shape and strength with exercise over a period of weeks or months. Nerves also recover from the mild or moderate degrees of damage likely in childbirth although the process of regaining strength after nerve injury is slow and may be incomplete. While the nerve supplying a muscle is out of action the muscle begins to waste from disuse, so the nerve must recover or regrow first and then the muscle must be built up by exercise. Badly stretched ligament does not heal well but the 'ligaments' supporting the urethra contain a substantial proportion of muscle and should recover better than other ligaments would do.

In many cases incontinence dates back to a pregnancy rather than to a birth although doctors do not know exactly what happens during pregnancy to cause it. We do know that hormones are produced in pregnancy which make ligaments more stretchy, and that joints are more vulnerable to injury as a result. The load of the pregnant uterus above a pelvic floor made slack by these hormones probably contributes to a harmful degree of stretch. There could also be damage directly by pressure on nerves or indirectly by pressure on blood vessels restricting the blood supply to some areas of muscle.

Straining to empty the bowel puts intense pressure on the pelvic floor muscles while they are relaxed and inhibits the contraction which should automatically follow defaecation. Continued as a habit over years, it contributes to muscle and nerve injury. Chronic coughing and obesity are additional factors. The pelvic floor muscles are notably thinner in fat women than in those of average build, and a number of specialist doctors have commented on the high proportion of their incontinent patients who are overweight.

There is a general loss of muscular strength in older people and the supporting muscles of the urinary system are affected along with the rest. Active exercise slows the process and it must be helpful to build up the muscles in the early and middle years to allow a greater safety margin for some inevitable attrition later.

All muscles atrophy if they are not used and strengthen if they are. The pelvic floor muscles have a sexual function as well as a supportive one, and one researcher[3] explained very coyly in 1963 that if incontinence began 'upon a change in sexual activity, such as loss of the husband might entail' it could be due to muscle atrophy from disuse. He was not so rude as to suggest appropriate remedial activity! I wouldn't rely on it anyway. Sex might help but it can hardly be essential; otherwise virgins would all be incontinent. Still, if you need an excuse . . .

Prolapse of the uterus or vagina is a separate consequence of poor pelvic support. It is not a direct cause of incontinence. An operation simply to correct uterine or vaginal prolapse will not in itself cure stress incontinence; it could even cause it. However, an operation for stress incontinence might be combined with an operation for prolapse. Prolapse of the bladder or urethra is more relevant although incontinence does not automatically follow from it. If your doctor says you have 'prolapse', ask him to explain exactly which part has prolapsed, and if surgery is suggested ask whether and how it is expected to improve your urinary symptoms. Enlargement of the uterus (unless it is absolutely massive) does not cause incontinence and therefore hysterectomy will not cure it.

## Disorders of Coordination

The nervous system oversees the whole operation of holding and releasing urine and harmonizes the action of the many muscles involved. Any injury or illness affecting the central nervous system (brain and spinal cord) or the peripheral nerves supplying the bladder, urethra or pelvic floor can produce urinary symptoms.

The peripheral nerves may be damaged in accidents, if the pelvis is fractured for instance, or during surgical operations, or as a result of childbearing. The central nervous system has substantial bony protection but it too is vulnerable in accidents which cause severe injuries to the back, neck or head. The loss of normal bladder control in people paralysed by spinal injuries is a particular problem; not only is it distressing in itself but it leaves the urinary tract susceptible to dangerous infections.

The central part of the coordinating system in the brain and spinal cord integrates information from several sources and initiates appropriate reactions. Playing such a pivotal role, it can produce practically any urinary symptom if it goes wrong. It depends on a sensory arm to gather and deliver the information and a motor arm to relay instructions to the muscles which finally produce the response. Disorders in the sensory or motor sections also give rise to a variety of symptoms.

If the sensory side of the control system is too responsive, the result is likely to be a sensation of urgency (and perhaps urge incontinence) when the bladder is only part full. Curiously, urgency and urge incontinence might also result if the sensory department is sluggish and fails to inform the conscious levels of the brain that the bladder is full before the lower levels of the spinal cord set off a reflex emptying contraction of the bladder muscle. It is sometimes suggested that this sort of sluggishness contributes to bedwetting, the sensation of bladder fullness being too weak to awaken the sleeper in time. Complete failure of the stretch sensors would allow the bladder to overfill and overflow.

The nerves on the motor side of the system serve the bladder, urethra and pelvic floor. The contractions of these muscles will be weakened or even abolished if the nerves supplying them are damaged. Reduced activity in the urethra and pelvic floor contributes to stress incontinence while paralysis of the bladder muscle precludes normal emptying and can cause overflow incontinence.

If the detrusor muscle of your bladder contracts at inappropriate times and without your wanting it to, there is some fault in the working of the coordinating system. The central controls are either setting off detrusor contractions in response to unusually mild provocation or failing to inhibit them in the normal way. All the same, it is convenient to talk of 'detrusor instability' and blame the behaviour on an 'unstable bladder'. In the same way, it is convenient to call the treatment in Chapter 8 a 'bladder training program' although it is largely directed towards improving the working of the control centre.

The idea of bladder instability has been around for a long time but it is equally plausible that a failure of central control might affect the urethral or pelvic floor muscles and cause 'urethral instability' or 'pelvic floor instability'. Inappropriate relaxation of these muscles allows urine leakage. If urethral relaxation accompanies an unstable bladder contraction, the result is more by way of a flood.

A disease like multiple sclerosis will produce varying symptoms according to which parts of the central nervous system have been affected. If areas connected with urinary control become involved, bladder problems become likely, and the same is true of other neurological disorders such as Parkinson's disease. Similarly, a stroke will disrupt bladder control if it happens to occur in an area of the brain with urinary responsibilities.

Strokes are more common in later years and, along with accumulated wear and tear on the brain, doubtless contribute to the increased prevalence of incontinence in older people. Strokes kill brain cells and new cells do not grow to replace them. However, it is a mistake to suppose that a bladder problem caused by a stroke will necessarily be with you for the rest of your life. Undamaged brain cells remain and they have a remarkable ability to take over new functions; it is a slow process but you do have a chance of relearning bladder control.

Epilepsy is in a different category. Between attacks, bladder control is normal but incontinence is not unusual during a major seizure when a tide of electrical activity sweeps across large sections of the brain. There is a suggestion that a similar mechanism accounts for some cases of giggle incontinence, with electrical activity spreading from a 'laughter centre' in the brain to a bladder control centre. There is no proof for this but doctors have treated at least one person successfully with a drug which curbs the spread of electrical activity[4].

It is impossible to say where the brain ends and the mind begins; philosophers have fought territorial disputes over the boundary for centuries. Still, there is no question that the states of your mind, your brain and your body are all closely interwoven, with influences going in both directions. Psychological stresses can disturb bladder control just as they can produce clear physical symptoms in many other parts of the body.

# Moving On

You cannot tell exactly what has gone wrong in your own body to produce your bladder problem without extensive tests. Even with all the tests, a doctor cannot always be perfectly sure what is at the root of your difficulty. Luckily, the three basic self-help treatments are effective in very many cases and you do not need to pinpoint the precise cause of the trouble in order to select the most appropriate of the three.

All the same, one of the questions you have probably whispered to yourself in the past is 'Why me?' Understanding something of how the urinary system works, and knowing what your symptoms are and when they started, you may be able to make quite a good guess at what has happened to cause your problem and that may make you feel better about it. Once you have had your guess, though, it is time to get on to the following chapters and take some action. To understand all may be to forgive all, but it certainly is not to cure all.

# Chapter 6

# STARTING YOUR SELF-HELP PROGRAM

Providing that you have eliminated cystitis as a cause of your difficulties, and have seen a doctor if necessary, the next few steps are the same whatever the problem you are aiming to overcome.

The very first thing to do is to make a definite decision that beating your bladder problem is important enough to you that you are prepared to see the self-help scheme through. Both bladder training and pelvic floor exercise require determination and persistence. There is absolutely no point in starting either treatment program with the idea of trying it out for a few weeks and seeing if it works. If you start half-heartedly and give up after a couple of weeks, you will get nowhere.

Once you have made the decision to help yourself, the next three steps are ABC — Assess, Begin and Continue.

Beginning is easy, but be ready to use every trick you know to bribe, threaten and cajole yourself into continuing long enough to see an improvement in your symptoms. You have a better chance of noticing a small improvement, and being encouraged by it to continue your good work, if you make a careful record of your state at the start. That is why it is so important to assess your condition before you begin working to improve it. The first part of this chapter tells you how.

Some other factors which may not appear at first sight to be related to your bladder problem could also be aggravating matters. You will need to assess whether any of these apply to you so that you can start putting them right. These questions are covered in the second part of the chapter.

The third part of the chapter is to point you towards the most appropriate self-help regime and help you into the right frame of mind to make a go of it.

# Sizing Up the Problem

The aim here is to have a good look at how your bladder behaves now and give yourself a baseline from which to measure progress.

For one week make a note every time you empty your bladder deliberately and every time you have an accident or have to make an urgent dash for the toilet. Notice roughly how large each leak was (a few drops, a spoonful, a flood) and what caused it. Each day count up how many leaks you had and how many times you deliberately emptied your bladder. If you used pads to absorb the urine keep track of how many you used each day or make a note of how often you had to change your pants.

If your only problem is stress incontinence it is not essential to measure the quantity of urine you pass, but if you are trying to overcome urgency, frequency, nocturia or anything else it is extremely helpful to know the volume you produce on each occasion. All you need is an ordinary kitchen-type measuring jug, as sold in all good hardware stores. There is no need to use disinfectants or take any special precautions; after use, simply tip the urine into the toilet, rinse the jug with water ready for next time and wash your hands as usual. Unless you are prepared to carry your jug everywhere you go, choose a day when you can stay at home and write down the volume of urine (in millilitres or fluid ounces) every time you empty your bladder in a 24-hour period.

You can draw up a chart to record all this but it is just as good to write it down as a list on ordinary paper. The important thing is to look at what really happens and not guess or try to remember what happened last week instead. And don't cheat! It may be depressing to realize just how many episodes of incontinence you have but you must have an accurate picture of your state at the start of your self-help program. After a few weeks it will be hard to remember exactly how you were to start with and you may improve so gradually that you won't notice until you compare with your original record. So however miserable this list of leaks and mishaps may seem, don't throw it away. It is the first step in your journey towards better bladder control.

Now you know how many leaks you have in a week it is time to have a close look at what causes them. Do you lose urine accidentally only if you are standing up, or can it happen in any position? Do you leak with very mild movements, or when you walk steadily, or with more vigorous activity like running or skipping? What about coughing, sneezing or laughing? Does your bladder have to be full or can you have accidents soon after you have been to the toilet? About how much urine do you lose each time? Make a note of this too and keep it with your week's record.

If you lose urine with fairly mild provocation, you will now have a very thorough idea of your starting level. You will know how many times a week or a day you have accidents, how large they are and what causes them. On the other hand, if you only lose urine with strenuous activity it is not very helpful to measure the number of leaks in a week because it just depends on how many times you exercise that vigorously. In this case you need to work out some other way of measuring your incontinence. For instance, if running is your trouble spot, keep a record each time you run of whether and how much you leak. Or if skipping is a particular problem, record how much urine you lose with a single jump or how many jumps you can do and still stay dry.

The next thing to look at is how frequently you are emptying your bladder deliberately. Don't guess. Go back to your week's record and look. A typical healthy woman empties her bladder 4 to 6 times a day. If you are emptying yours 7 or more times each day you should stop to think why.

The likeliest reason is that you are drinking a great deal of liquid. In this case you are bound to produce a lot of urine and since your bladder can only hold a certain amount you will be forced to empty it frequently. There is nothing necessarily unhealthy about drinking so much but it does make regular trips to the loo inevitable. You simply need to decide which you want more, the drink or the time away from the toilet.

If your favourite drink is tea, coffee or cola, the problem is a little more complicated. As well as all the water in them, these drinks contain caffeine and other stimulants. Caffeine is a diuretic which means that it promotes urine production. It also affects the nerves in your body, including the nerves which control your bladder, so it may well make bladder control more difficult. It is not very likely that this is the only cause of your incontinence but it could be making it worse. It would be sensible to cut the caffeine out of your diet, at least for a few weeks, and see if it helps. Switch to decaffeinated brands of tea and coffee or choose other drinks altogether. Make the change gradually if your body has been accustomed to having a generous supply of caffeinated drinks.

Another possible cause for constant trips to the loo is pregnancy. So many women have urinary frequency when they are pregnant that it is considered normal. There is no need to do anything about it except wait for the birth. Just make sure that you don't keep the habit of frequent voiding after your baby is born.

If you are emptying your bladder very often, before it even feels full, perhaps you are trying to avoid leaks by keeping your bladder permanently empty. This is a very bad habit to get into. It is not very effective and in the long run it is more than likely to make the problem worse.

Firstly, it undermines your confidence in the ability of your bladder to hold a normal amount of urine. Then you find yourself voiding at shorter and shorter intervals and in the end this can be even more of a nuisance than the incontinence you started with. Secondly, the muscles with which you voluntarily stop the flow of urine are not being made to work, so they are likely to become weaker. The weaker they are, the less they are able to prevent urine leakage. Thirdly, if you never allow your bladder to fill in the normal way, it may become very sensitive to stretching and contract in response, unlike a normal bladder which remains relaxed while it fills so that the pressure inside does not rise very much. In other words you are encouraging your bladder to become unstable. You have enough to deal with already without adding bladder instability as a further source of difficulty.

You must give up the idea of emptying your bladder at every opportunity and start allowing it a more natural cycle of filling and emptying. Wait until your bladder signals that it is full before you consider emptying it. If this simple approach does not give you reasonable intervals between visits to the toilet, see Chapter 8 for a stricter regime of bladder training.

If you are not pregnant, not drinking huge amounts of liquid, not emptying your bladder as a pre-emptive measure and do not have cystitis, you probably have a problem of frequency which needs to be tackled head-on using the scheme in Chapter 8.

Holding on to your urine so that you empty your bladder much less often than the normal 4-6 times a day is not advisable either. Bladder infections can get a grip more easily when urine is held in your body for long periods. There is also a suggestion that habitually holding very large volumes of urine could reduce the bladder's normal sensitivity to stretch which is a key element in healthy bladder control. Overstretching the bladder might even damage the closure mechanism at the bladder neck.

If you only visit the toilet two or three times a day, make a conscious decision to go more often, either when you first feel an urge or at predetermined times. Godec[1] found that his patients reduced their incontinence markedly by emptying their bladders at fixed 2-hour intervals but I would suggest an interval of three or four hours as closer to a normal voiding pattern.

# Some Related Questions

You have taken stock of your situation now and you know exactly what scale of problem you are aiming to overcome. The next step is to ask some more questions about yourself and the ways you have already responded to your incontinence. You may be making matters worse without realizing it. The first four questions are important whatever your difficulty; the remaining five are especially relevant if you suffer from stress incontinence.

# 1 Are you drinking a reasonable amount?

A reasonable amount means three to four pints (six large mugs or ten cups) of watery drinks per day. If you are drinking less in the hope of leaking less you are doing yourself no good at all. It is neither possible nor helpful to keep your bladder permanently empty. If you are drinking very small quantities you are giving your kidneys a hard time and increasing your chances of developing a bladder infection into the bargain. Also, your urine will be very concentrated so it may irritate the urethra and give you a misleadingly urgent desire to empty your bladder.

Err on the side of drinking too much rather than too little, and if it seems a bit cock-eyed to produce more urine when you have a problem in holding it just remember that practice makes perfect. You want perfect bladder control so you need plenty of urine to practise on!

# 2 Do you use tampons to prevent leaks or pads to absorb urine?

Some women find that wearing a firmly fitting tampon prevents urine leakage because it gives some support to the bladder and urethra. If tampons work for you it is quite sensible to use them occasionally, maybe a couple of times a week while you exercise. It will cause no problems and it is much pleasanter than having to use a pad to soak up the urine. However, it is not a good idea to wear tampons all the time. It is the job of your pelvic muscles to support your internal organs; if you use tampons to do the job instead then the muscles will get lazier and weaker in just the same way that your abdominal muscles do if you rely on support girdles to hold your tummy in.

Pads are different from tampons because they have no direct physical effect on your bladder or pelvic muscles so the question whether or when to use them is much more personal. If you know you are certain to leak at some particular time, during the keep-fit class for instance, then the decision about pads for that occasion is trivial; you need to wear them. It is all the rest of the time when you only think you might leak that the question becomes tricky.

You need to build up your self-confidence as much as possible so that you can approach your self-help program with the determination it needs. The more you let your incontinence affect your activities, the more it will undermine your confidence, so you should behave as normally as possible — wear normal clothes, go out, talk to your friends, get on with your work, make your plans, do your usual activities. Wearing normal clothes means not wearing pads. Once you start wearing them all the time you are on your way to accepting your incontinence as a permanent fact in your life, and that is not a good starting point from which to overcome it. On the other hand, if you are absolutely terrified of leaking you will do better to use pads sometimes so that you can keep up your other activities and free your mind to think about something other than your bladder. Extreme anxiety itself makes the bladder more difficult to control so you may even find that using a pad to take away the fear of leaking actually enables you to stay dry.

In general it is best to wear pads as little as possible. If you have got very used to wearing them all the time, start by leaving them off for a short time in a place where a leak would be an inconvenience, not a disaster. The more time you spend pad-free, the more confidence you will develop in your own ability to control your bladder. As your control and confidence grow, aim to use smaller pads and use them on fewer occasions until finally you can dispense with them altogether.

## 3 Are you taking any medicines?

Some drugs are intended to affect your urinary system; many others may influence bladder control as a side-effect. If your incontinence began or worsened when you started taking any medicines, talk to your doctor about it. There may be an alternative which does not affect you in the same way.

## 4 Did the incontinence start or get worse at the menopause?

If so, it is particularly worth seeing your doctor because the symptoms may be related to the hormonal changes going on in your body and hormone replacement could be a real help.

You should still do the exercises explained in Chapter 7 as well. If the menopause has made the lining of your urethra thinner so that it does not form a watertight seal so easily as it used to, you cannot afford to lose any of the strength in the muscles supporting and controlling it. These muscles tend to weaken as you get older and the only way to help them keep their strength is to exercise them.

## 5 Do you have a constant cough?

Coughing will make you leak of course, which is annoying, but, more significantly, it will renew the injury to your pelvic floor muscles. Every cough produces a sudden sharp rise in the pressure in your abdomen. If your pelvic muscles are strong this pressure will have little effect on them but while they are weak it will make them stretch suddenly. Sudden stretching can damage both the muscles and the nerves that supply them. A chronic cough is never healthy and it will spoil your chances of overcoming stress incontinence. If you have a persistent cough, see your doctor: if you cough because you smoke the treatment is in your own hands.

## 6 Do you strain down to empty your bowels?

Straining is a very damaging habit. Like coughing, it raises the pressure in your abdomen and, worse still, if you are straining to open your bowels you are raising the pressure at just the time when the pelvic muscles are relaxed and so most vulnerable to stretching. There is evidence that persistent straining causes injury to the nerves supplying various pelvic muscles including the sphincters and it is implicated as a cause of both urinary and faecal incontinence.

If your straining is just a habit, stop it. When your bowel is full it will naturally empty itself; you need only relax and wait for the muscular activity of the rectum to push the contents out. Do not try to hurry it and especially do not insist that you should empty your bowels at fixed intervals such as every day.

If you strain because you are really constipated, adjust your diet. Drink more water and eat more fibre (fruit, vegetables, wholemeal bread etc.). If the problem remains after a few weeks on this regime, see your doctor.

You should also see your doctor if you need to strain to empty your bladder.

## 7 Do you do a lot of heavy lifting?

Lifting has a similar effect on your pelvic muscles to coughing as it raises abdominal pressure. Until your muscles are strong enough to resist it, that rise in pressure will stretch and possibly damage them. Whenever you can, avoid heavy lifting altogether. If you have a job like looking after a toddler which makes lifting unavoidable, protect your pelvic floor as much as possible. Pull up the muscles as for the pelvic floor exercises in Chapter 7 before you start to lift and move steadily, not jerkily. Remember to protect your back too.

## 8 Are you overweight?

Being overweight increases the pressure on your bladder and on your pelvic floor. The greater the pressure, the more likely you are to leak. If you are overweight, just getting out of bed could put as much pressure on your bladder as running does for a slimmer, more agile, person[2]. You will have a much better chance of achieving full bladder control if you lose weight. There is so much advice available on how to reduce your weight that it would be pointless to repeat it here. Just remember what a very good reason you now have to stick to your diet. The fatter you are, the slimmer your chances of success in beating your bladder problem.

## 9 Do you wear a support girdle, corsets or very tight clothes?

Throw them out. They increase the pressure on your bladder and make you more likely to leak. They will also make your abdominal muscles flabby. The only healthy way to have a flat tummy is to tone up your muscles by exercise. Begin gently if they are very much out of condition; the postnatal exercises issued to new mothers are a good starting point.

# Getting Ready to Go

Now that you have made the decision to help yourself and have done a thorough assessment of your situation, you are very nearly ready to start your self-treatment in earnest.

If you suffer purely from stress incontinence, you will be following the regime of pelvic floor exercise in Chapter 7. If your main bugbear is frequency, urgency or a related difficulty, the primary treatment is the bladder training program in Chapter 8. However, you should also consider strengthening your pelvic floor muscles by exercise. This will not affect the sense of urgency directly but you will be better able to cut off the flow of urine and limit the scale of any leak. If you have stress incontinence in addition to frequency or urgency, you will have to use both bladder training and pelvic floor exercise.

It is too much to start on the two treatment schedules at the same time, so begin with one and add in the other a few weeks later. It is not critical which one you choose for starters and both have their advantages. If you begin with the exercises for stress incontinence, after a few weeks your pelvic muscles will be beginning to gain a little more strength and will be in better shape for their part in the work of bladder training. On the other hand, if you start with bladder training you will see the first signs of progress earlier and this may give you some useful encouragement to continue.

For bedwetting or other forms of incontinence, read Chapter 9 or 10 before you go back to 7 or 8.

If beating your bladder problem is a sea crossing, and choosing your treatment is finding the right boat, you are just about ready to set sail now. You have studied the maps to see where you are, you have plotted out your course and you have checked the rigging to make sure that everything is set up to work as smoothly as possible. All that is left before you pull up the anchor is to clear the decks.

The first unnecessary burden to throw overboard is secrecy. Guard your privacy, of course, and choose carefully whom you tell, but do talk to somebody. If your family would not be sympathetic, tell a friend. If your friend is a woman with children, the chances are that she has had (or still has) the same difficulty herself even if she has never given a hint of it! If you can't find a suitable friend, find a sympathetic doctor or a professional counsellor.

Next, waste no time wondering whether your craft will float. It may look ramshackle but it is the only one available for a singlehanded crossing and many women have steered a successful course across this stretch of water in boats just like it. Your chances of success are very good if you follow your schedule diligently, but what is even more certain is that if you do not take action your problem will remain or get worse.

The last two things to clear out of the way are anxiety and obsession. If you cannot actually throw them over the side, at least get them stowed away and lashed down so that if the going gets choppy you won't find them sliding around on the decks of your mind to trip you up.

Anxiety and unhappiness have a definite effect on bladder control. They are likely to make your problem worse and they are certain to make it harder for you to concentrate on the treatment.

Be honest about whether any unhappiness you have is really due to your bladder problem. A course of bladder training or pelvic floor exercise will not put everything right if there are other things in your life worrying or upsetting you. You are already doing something positive about your incontinence; try to do the same for your other worries. If you cannot see the root of the problem or do anything practical to tackle it, ask a doctor or counsellor for help. Depression can be treated and you can learn techniques to overcome anxiety.

If you are anxious because you are afraid of leaking through a pad, get some advice about better pads. Many shops sell pads intended for use during periods and while these work well enough for very small amounts of urine, pads designed for incontinence are very much better. They come in various sizes and some are made with a super-absorbent gel so they can soak up a surprising amount of urine without being very bulky and without feeling very wet. Some have an adhesive strip to stick to your own pants while others are made to slip into a pouch in special 'pouch pants'.

Usually both pads and pants are on display on the open shelves so you need not actually ask for them, but if you want advice about the different types the assistant, or perhaps the pharmacist, will be helpful. You can even buy incontinence pads by mail order. So long as you change pads regularly there will be no noticeable smell from them. Spray-on deodorants are not necessary; they may actually irritate the area and so make matters worse.

As for obsession, do not confuse it with determination. You may have to do your pelvic floor exercise for one minute every hour, for instance, and that will take determination. What you do not have to do is think about your bladder for the other fifty-nine minutes! Do what your schedule requires and for the rest of the time get on with your normal life. And don't keep looking for signs of progress every half day; that is obsessive too and it will only demoralize you.

At first, just concentrate on following your regime and congratulate yourself on the fact that you are taking positive action. Then, when you do start to make progress, focus on what you have achieved, not on what you still have to achieve. Be pleased when you are dry for a longer spell than you used to be, or dare to do something that you would not have done before.

Above all, reject the idea that because you have a bladder problem you are weak or helpless or somehow inferior to all those people whom you suppose to have perfect bladder control. It is not your fault that you suffered from incontinence in the first place, but it is to your credit that you are doing something about it. In fact, every day that you complete your self-help program you are proving just what a strong-minded character you are!

# Chapter 7

# STRESS INCONTINENCE

The core of the self-treatment for stress incontinence is pelvic floor exercise. Before you start on it, you should have checked whether you need to see a doctor, assessed the scale of the problem and made a start on sorting out anything which could be making it worse. These points are covered in Chapters 3 and 6.

Strengthening your pelvic floor muscles by exercise is intended to have two effects. It will make them better able to contract actively and help shut off the urethra during stressful events such as sneezing. It should also make them larger and firmer so that they provide more support to the bladder and urethra even when you are relaxed.

You cannot expect results from this exercise in a short time any more than you could train up for a marathon or recover from a knee injury in a short time. On the other hand, you would never attempt to train for a marathon if you thought that running would have no effect on your fitness so before you go into the program of pelvic muscle exercise you will want to know the answers to two questions—will it work and how long will it take?

## Will it Work and How Long will it Take?

The idea of pelvic floor exercise became popular following the work of Kegel. [10,11] He invented a device to measure the squeeze produced in the vagina when the pelvic floor muscles are contracted and his patients used this to help them do the exercise correctly. Exercising for about twenty minutes, three times a day, Kegel reported that all the women with simple stress incontinence were much improved, usually within eight weeks. Women with more severe or complex difficulties sometimes took as much as a year to achieve success.

Since then, many other workers have recommended pelvic floor exercise and, as the treatment has become more widespread, many slightly different versions have come into use. There has been a tendency over the years to drop the use of the measuring device and to suggest exercising not in three long sessions but in a larger number of short ones. The form of pelvic floor exercise described in this book is in line with the usual practice of the last ten years.

Few of the doctors who treat incontinence with exercise today would claim a success rate quite as high as that reported by Kegel in the early 1950s. Perhaps women were more tolerant of minor inconvenience forty years ago, or perhaps Kegel was so enthusiastic about his new technique that he overestimated the degree of improvement in some of his patients. However, these possible objections do not apply to the recent reports by independent workers who confirm that pelvic floor exercise is a useful treatment for the majority of women with stress incontinence.

In six studies published between 1983 and 1988,[2,3,4,7,19,22] a total of 174 women used pelvic floor exercise for up to three months. 70 per cent of them were cured or improved. In the three studies[2,7,19] which gave information about cure and improvement separately, 40 per cent of the 114 women considered themselves to be completely cured and in two of those studies[7,19] the cure was confirmed by objective evidence.

A cure rate of 40 per cent and an improvement rate of 70 per cent is very good from a doctor's point of view, particularly for a treatment which has no significant side-effects. Looked at pessimistically from the other side, though, it implies that 30 per cent, or one in three, of the women entering the programs were not helped by exercise. In fact, such pessimism is unjustified because a common cause of lack of progress was failure to follow the exercise regime faithfully.

Jones and Kegel,[9] for instance, found that half the patients who did not reach a good result by exercise were women who gave up after less than two months. For those who complete a three-month exercise program, the chance of success is higher than the average in these reports, and the chances are probably higher still if exercise is maintained for longer.

In these recent studies, the length of the treatment varied from four weeks to three months. Both Benvenuti's and Castleden's groups[2,4] found some improvement within two weeks of starting exercise which is too short a time for the muscles to gain much in strength. Presumably the women gained some benefit as soon as they learnt the trick of contracting the pelvic floor to prevent leaks during short stresses such as coughs. By contrast, Jones and Kegel[9] found that almost half of the women who eventually achieved success on their exercise program showed no progress in the first two months, and Mandelstam[13] felt that it could take as much as three weeks before a woman even develops a definite awareness of the pelvic muscle contraction.

There is little well-organized information on this question of how long it takes before symptoms first begin to show some signs of diminishing, and probably there is a great deal of variation from one woman to another. As a rough guide you can hope to see some improvement after about six weeks of intensive exercise, but you should expect to keep on with the treatment for three months or more.

Pelvic floor exercise is an appropriate treatment to try whether you are young or old, whether you have mild or severe symptoms and whether you have had them for weeks or for decades. Kegel[11] was particularly struck by the success of some his older patients, in their seventies and not in good general health. On a six-week exercise program[22] older women were less successful than others but this probably only means that they needed longer to reach their goal because age had no bearing on the outcome after a nine-week[5] or three-month[7] treatment. Similarly, women with more severe symptoms at the start were less likely to achieve complete continence after six or nine weeks, but after three months they were equally as successful as others. In the three-month study, women whose bladder problems had lasted for more than three years made less progress than those whose difficulties had begun more recently although, again, this may only mean that a long-established weakness takes longer to overcome.

Conscientious pelvic floor exercise usually works well. If you have tried it before without success ask yourself whether you really did it long enough and seriously enough. Advocates of pelvic floor exercise tend to overemphasize its simplicity and effectiveness and underplay the effort and time required. Perhaps you were misled into believing that it would produce dramatic results quickly and gave up when it did not do so. This time, resolve to follow the program unwaveringly for three months and you will have an excellent chance of regaining continence.

# What to Do

There are two parts to the treatment program. The most important part, repeated pelvic floor contractions or 'pelvic lifts', can be done anywhere, anytime, and I will explain it in detail later. The second part you must do with a full bladder.

Next time you feel a need to empty your bladder, delay for a few minutes. You have probably done this unthinkingly hundreds of times before but this time notice what you do with your muscles to hold on to your urine. If you can delay without apparently doing anything, wait until your bladder is really full and hold on, or try holding on for a few moments after you have sat down on the toilet. You will automatically tense up your pelvic floor muscles to do this and you should be able to feel the difference when you relax them to allow urine to flow. The main point of this part of the exercise is to become aware of the muscles so that you can learn to contract them at will.

There is no need to wait until you are bursting every time before you empty your bladder but do avoid visiting the toilet at every opportunity. You may remember from Chapter 5 that there are two types of muscle involved in supporting and closing the urethra, smooth and striped, and you want both to be as strong as possible. You will strengthen the striped muscle by deliberate exercise but you cannot do the same for the smooth muscle as it is not under direct conscious control. However, both sorts contract by reflex action when your bladder fills, so delaying urination gives you a way of making the smooth muscle work. It also helps to discourage bladder instability.

Do not get carried away with the idea of holding on to your urine. It is not healthy to overstretch your bladder any more than it is healthy to keep it always empty. As a general guide, 400-500 ml (14-17 fluid ounces) is a typical volume of urine to produce when the bladder feels very full. If you are prone to cystitis it is important to empty your bladder regularly so you will have to drink plenty if you want it to fill to capacity.

The next exercise to be done with a full bladder is to stop the stream of urine after you have started it. Do not be surprised or worried if you find it difficult or impossible at first. Plenty of perfectly continent women cannot stop their streams to order either. It is not an important skill in itself but it is a useful exercise as you can see the effect at the time and so learn to contract the right muscles to close the urethra.

To begin with, try stopping the stream early on (before it really gets going) or as it slows down towards the end. Try to relax all your other muscles, especially tummy and buttocks, while you pull up and squeeze around your anus, vagina and urethra. The stream should slow down or stop. If it speeds up it will be because you are tensing other muscles at the same time. Hold the contraction for several seconds, then let go again. If there is still urine flowing, slow it or stop it twice more.

Take particular care to empty your bladder completely after this exercise. If you stop the stream effectively you may lose the feeling of desire to void even while there is still urine in your bladder and, left there, this would make infection more likely. Use the exercise only occasionally if you are prone to cystitis. Be sparing with it also if you are following a bladder training program as it is important to know that you have emptied your bladder completely so that you do not give yourself any excuse to break your schedule. When you are emptying your bladder immediately before planned exercise, release the urine all in one go so that the least possible amount is left behind.

The stop stream exercise is just that — an exercise, not a test. Do not feel bad because you cannot stop in a fraction of a second as most men can, feel good because you are working the muscles. It may take a long time before you feel you are getting anywhere but carry on practising once or twice a day. As you strengthen you will gradually become able to stop more quickly, completely and confidently.

When you have overcome your incontinence, or learned to stop your flow midstream in less than a second, give up doing the exercise regularly. You are effectively producing a temporary obstruction to the flow of urine and we do know that long-term obstruction can lead to bladder instability (which reverses when the obstruction is removed). Stop stream training has been widely used without ill effect but, when the exercise is no longer needed, it is a sensible precaution to return to uninterrupted emptying.

The key element to pelvic floor exercise is the 'pelvic lift', a contraction of the pelvic floor muscles which lifts the perineum and tends to close the urethra, vagina and anus; it is the movement you use in the stop stream exercise and it also helps to stop bowel gas escaping. You may already be aware of these muscles and able to contract them at will or, like many women, you may need to learn to contract them before you can start active exercise. It takes time to learn because the movement is small and not easily detectable (especially at first while the muscles are weak) so be persistent and use whichever you find most helpful of the images offered below. As you carry on practising, the movement will become stronger and you will be able to feel it more easily.

Pull your pubic bone and your tailbone together, as if you were tucking your tail between your legs. (In animals with tails, this is what the pelvic floor muscles actually do.) At the same time, lift your perineum up into your body like a drawbridge or a lift moving up in a lift shaft. Imagine that you have an attack of diarrhoea, an urgent desire to empty your bladder or a need to release bowel gas which must be resisted at all costs. Remember which muscles you tense in the stop stream exercise and work the same ones now.

Do not bother trying to contract the muscles around your anus separately from those around your vagina and urethra. You might manage weak contractions of the individual parts but with strong contractions, and you need the strongest contractions possible, they all work together. Do not hold your breath and do not cross your legs, or tense your tummy or buttocks. The relevant muscles are well above the perineal skin, connecting your pubic bone to your tailbone, and this is where you should feel them stiffening.

Check that you are making the right movement by looking or feeling. With a mirror you will see the perineum lifting very slightly and, less importantly, the vagina and anus closing up. You can also feel the lift with a cupped hand between your legs or a finger resting lightly on the skin between the vagina and anus. If you are not sure that you are feeling in the right place, put your hand in position and bear down or strain gently. The perineum will bulge down. Now try lifting it up. In general, avoid activities which make the perineum bulge.

To feel the pelvic floor muscles more directly, place a finger or two (clean, of course) in your vagina and do a pelvic lift. There is a squeeze and a lift, and the front wall of the vagina is pulled into a curve behind the pubic bone. If you press your finger against the side of the vagina about half a finger's length inside, where the pelvic floor muscles pass by, you can feel them become firmer when you pull up. You can also try this squeezing on your partner's penis; he may enjoy it occasionally but he will not appreciate your pestering him every time to tell you how strong a squeeze you managed.

Hold the contraction as hard as you can for five seconds, then relax for five seconds before repeating it. Especially in the early days, the muscles are liable to relax themselves during the five seconds of holding so try to squeeze a bit harder still with each second. The muscle fatigues easily so there is no point trying to hold for longer periods, certainly not until you can manage five seconds easily, but it is essential to lift as high and squeeze as hard as you can. Exercise only strengthens muscles if they are made to work harder than normal and, since you are not giving your pelvic floor muscles an external load to work against, you are relying on your willpower to make sure they work hard enough.

Do the exercise in sessions of six lifts which will take one minute. Do it frequently and in various positions. Lying on your back or side with your legs bent at the hip and knee is good, particularly in the beginning, because it helps you to avoid tensing your buttocks and it allows the muscle to move more freely as it is working against less weight. Standing with your legs apart is good because it gives the muscle more of a load to work against. The standing position is also useful because, even if you cannot feel the lift very clearly, you will be able to tell that you did it correctly by the feeling of your perineum flopping down again afterwards.

Using a variety of positions has two advantages. It makes the exercise marginally less boring and it allows the muscle to work in all its ranges of movement. However, the most important thing is to do the exercise often enough (an absolute minimum of ten minutes a day) so use whatever positions let you fit it conveniently into your day.

# Sticking to the Program for a Day

The pelvic floor exercise must be done many times over. Do six lifts in a minute and count up the number of minutes you do each day to use as your score. Start by aiming for fifteen minutes per day and work up as your muscles gain strength and you get into the habit of slotting the exercise into your routine.

It is sensible to split the exercise into a number of sessions because the muscles tire easily, especially when you are just starting, and although you have to work them into overload there is no benefit in working them into exhaustion. Most workers suggest doing short blocks of exercise very frequently but when Kegel first reported the method he recommended his patients to do three sessions per day, each fifteen to twenty minutes long, and they progressed equally well. I cannot tell you whether it is more (or less, or equally) effective to use many short sessions or a few longish ones because no-one has done a proper study to find out. What I can tell you is that, however you arrange it, you should aim to do a total of fifteen minutes or more. The most popular pattern is to spread this through the day in blocks of a minute each. Divide it between at least three separate sessions in any case.

Luckily, you can do your pelvic lifts while you are doing other things so it is not too difficult to fit them into a busy day. Make a habit of doing some whenever you have the chance — while you are cleaning your teeth, waiting in queues, washing up, watching television and so on — and you will soon build up a useful number without taking up any spare time at all. The movement is all inside your body so no-one watching will notice anything and you can do them absolutely anywhere.

Various schemes have been devised to help you remember to do your exercises often enough during the day. One method is to do a minute of exercise on the hour, every hour. That will suit you if you like to have a detailed program and if you will be in a position to do them at those exact times. Choose a different system if you resent having to keep one eye on the clock (a constant reminder of the problem you are tackling) or if the hour always seems to come up at a point when you cannot do the exercise because you are running for a bus or talking to a client.

Another method is to place stickers in strategic points around the house or around your workplace and do a minute of exercise whenever you see one. Again, this works well if you actually notice the stickers (in my experience they become invisible after a few days) and if you really stop and exercise each time. Thinking 'Oh, yes, I must do my exercises' as you rush past is no substitute.

The third alternative is to choose fifteen or so unavoidable activities and do a set of exercises with each one. For example, if you do a minute of pelvic lifts every time you clean your teeth, every time you have a meal or a snack, every time you go to the toilet and every time you switch on the radio or television, you will have done ten to fifteen minutes of exercise by the end of the day with no further effort.

If you have a very haphazard lifestyle, try this last idea. Put a piece of string or a knitting row counter in your pocket. Do a set of exercises whenever you have a spare moment and tie a knot in the string or move the counter on by one. Then forget the whole business until your next spare moment. At the end of the day you will know how many minutes you have done and you will hardly have had to think about it at all. This method combines very well with the previous one.

If you have a regular exercise program already, pull up your pelvic floor during each movement. You will not be holding the lift for five seconds but it all adds up to a worthwhile amount of exercise and it helps to protect the pelvic muscles during movements like sit-ups which put a strain on them. However, it cannot protect them completely if your pelvic floor is very weak or if your exercise schedule is very strenuous. In either of these cases, you should avoid exercises which put a strain on your pelvic floor for a couple of months or so until you have built up its strength to match the strength of the rest of your body. Do the pelvic lift before coughing, sneezing or lifting heavy weights as well to reduce the chance of leaking and to protect the muscles from stretching.

Keep a record every day of how many minutes of pelvic floor exercise you have done. Set a target and award yourself a pat on the back when you reach it. As time goes on, aim to complete more sets each day.

Do not deceive yourself with any nonsense about not having enough time to carry out the exercises. If you really want to overcome your incontinence, fifteen minutes a day is a remarkably small price and it is not even fifteen minutes doing that and nothing else. What else are you doing while you clean your teeth after all? Besides, it very soon becomes a habit to exercise in odd minutes throughout the day, and the more habitual it is, the less time and trouble it seems to take.

Yes, of course it is tiresome having to remember the exercises, but do not turn them into more of a chore than they really are by thinking miserably about your incontinence all the time you are doing them. When you do other sorts of exercise, you surely don't make yourself miserable with thoughts of obesity or heart disease, so why treat this differently? It too is exercise you are doing to become fully fit, every session you do gets you a little closer to your goal and you can feel pleased with yourself every time simply for making the effort.

# Sticking to the Program for Three Months

The first two or three days of the schedule are easy, like the first couple of days of a new diet. There is a glow of optimism and self-satisfaction in the fact that you are taking action. After a few days the glow wears off, you feel as if you have been exercising diligently for weeks and you begin to wonder why your incontinence has not improved yet. And you need to keep going for another three months at least!

Your daily records are essential at this point to remind you how long you have really been in training and how well you are doing in carrying out the program. For the first few weeks, concentrate solely on completing your target number of minutes of exercise each day and each week. If you are susceptible to bribery, bribe yourself with some little reward for each target achieved, and think about your incontinence as little as possible.

It would obviously be easier to keep up your motivation if you could see some definite sign of progress. Forty years ago Kegel's patients used a 'perineometer' in the vagina to measure the strength of the squeeze from the pelvic floor muscles but you can do equally well without such a device. Use either a mirror or a finger instead (as described on page 76) to check that you are using the right muscles for the exercise.

However weak it is, within four weeks of starting the program you should be aware of some contraction when you try to do a pelvic lift. If not, approach a doctor for help because all your efforts will get you nowhere until you can make the appropriate muscles respond to your instructions. You should not get back-ache, belly-ache or buttock-ache from these exercises. If you do, you are working the wrong muscles. Try to relax everywhere else and feel the tension only in the pelvic floor.

You may be able to tell that the pelvic floor muscles are responding more strongly within a few weeks, but do not look for any improvement in your symptoms so soon. They may even get worse at first if you start by trying too severe an exercise program, because the muscles will be fatigued. If this happens, ease off on the exercise for a while and build up again gradually.

After about six weeks you can sensibly start to use whatever test procedure you chose when you worked out your baseline in Chapter 6. If you want to make the test as fair as possible you should do it at about the same time of day, at about the same interval after your last visit to the toilet and, if your period affects your bladder control, at about the same stage of your menstrual cycle each time.

Choose your test so that it has a chance of showing the first small signs of progress. If your stress incontinence is severe, for example, use a short walk or a day's urinary diary as your test, not a minute of skipping. You can always make the test more demanding once you are regularly dry on the easier one. Do not test so often that the change is too small to see; once a month is enough. Keep a record of your success on tests too, along with your record of exercise done, so that you can compare from month to month.

It is tremendously encouraging when you first begin to see some improvement, and it gives a well-earned boost to your determination to keep going. There will also be times when progress seems slow and, of course, it is even more important to carry on with the exercises then. Whether or not it seems to be going well, stick at it for a full three months. Pelvic floor exercise is a siege tactic in the fight against incontinence, and your most important attribute is your persistence.

# Reviewing Progress

After three months many women will notice a substantial improvement and it is a fair time to review progress.

If you are happy with the state you have reached, you can stop exercising so assiduously and cut out the stop stream exercise altogether. Keep up a small amount of pelvic floor exercise, about five minutes a day, indefinitely to keep the muscles in good shape and prevent any relapse. If you notice your symptoms returning at any time, increase your exercise level again immediately to control them.

If you have improved but still have some way to go, keep on with the exercises. It takes more than three months to build up from a low level, particularly from injury, to reach peak fitness in any physical activity. Your pelvic floor muscles are no different from other muscles in this respect so you can expect to continue to improve if you continue to train.

You may need to increase your exercise level if you made some progress initially but feel that you have now reached a plateau. Just as a regular three-mile run will tone you up enormously but will not fit you to run a marathon, fifteen or twenty minutes of pelvic floor exercise may be enough to ease your symptoms but not cure them. You can vary the program by trying to hold the pelvic lift for longer than five seconds or by putting in lots of shorter lifts, but it is basically a matter of doing many more contractions and doing them all as strongly as possible.

Do not despair if you do not seem to have made much progress at all yet. Success may be just around the corner! Roughly a third of the women who finally achieved a good result under the guidance of Jones and Kegel[9] needed between two and six months to do so, and only half achieved their goal in less than two months.

First, check that when you try to do the pelvic lift you are actually lifting the perineum and squeezing inside the vagina, not just at the entrance. If there is some movement, even if it is very small, you are doing the exercise correctly and if you keep on with it the muscles will eventually increase in strength. A doctor or physiotherapist could confirm that you are working the right muscles and give you some moral support, but they are unlikely to do more at this stage. If you cannot feel any movement at all, seek medical advice. You may be able to learn the proper contraction with personal help, or by using a perineometer or electrical stimulation.

After six months, most people will feel cured or very much improved. If so, you can reduce your exercise level to about five minutes a day for maintenance or increase your efforts for further improvement. If you are not happy with your progress, see your doctor. It is still possible that exercise will work for you (occasionally it may take longer than six months, particularly if there has been damage to the nerves or if the muscles have been unused for a long time and atrophied) but you deserve at least some more personal support and probably some more detailed investigation.

Make sure that your doctor understands that you have done pelvic floor exercises faithfully for however long it is, otherwise he will probably just advise you to exercise for three months and come back if there is no change. You have already done all that and now you should have more help. More help does not necessarily mean surgery; it means first of all more investigation, then advice and discussion of the possibilities.

Do not feel that you must accept any particular treatment if you do not want it and, if you refuse a treatment, do not feel that you wasted the doctor's time. It is his job to find out exactly what is wrong and explain what options there are, and it is your job to choose between the options. The help offered will depend on where you live, as some areas have specialist facilities not available in others, and the specialist doctors have different ideas from each other too.

# Alternatives
## Cone therapy

If you wanted to strengthen your arm muscles, you would exercise them against a load by lifting weights. Cone therapy applies the same principle to pelvic floor exercise. You would place a weighted cone inside the vagina for two fifteen-minute exercise periods each day and contract your pelvic floor muscles to keep it in place. As the muscles strengthened, you would use heavier cones. Since the use of weights is so well-tried in the exercise of other muscles, this is a very logical and promising idea.

In two recent studies,[16,17] about 20 per cent of the women who kept up the exercise for just one month considered themselves completely cured and a further 50 per cent had improved, an overall improvement rate of about 70 per cent. By using ordinary pelvic floor exercise after the month with cones, the women improved their symptoms even further. However, cone treatment is quite a new technique and it will take time for doctors to test it further before it becomes widely available.

## Biofeedback

Biofeedback simply means letting you know what your body is doing so that you can learn to make it do what you want. Feeling the squeeze in the vagina with a finger is the simplest form of bio-feedback for pelvic muscle exercise. A slightly more sophisticated method is to use a vaginal pressure meter ('perineometer'). More elaborate schemes still (not in widespread use) involve several simultaneous pressure measurements. These devices may well make it easier to learn the correct muscle contraction, and no doubt they increase motivation, but they do not do the exercise for you. In the end your success still depends on your own efforts.

## Electrotherapy

There are various forms of electrical therapy but, in common with exercise, they have the aim of stimulating the muscles through the nerves. Unlike exercise, this kind of therapy does not require conscious effort, but it does require visits to a clinic and the use of specialist equipment. The position of the electrodes and the frequency and strength of the current need to be carefully adjusted so the electrical devices advertised in magazines for home use are not likely to work well.

Most of the studies on electrical therapy use pelvic floor exercise as part of the treatment. The overall success rate is not very different from that obtained by exercise alone and you could not expect any benefits to be maintained without continuing exercise after your course of electrical treatment was over. However, electrotherapy could be useful if you were having difficulty in learning to contract your pelvic floor muscles. You might find it easier once you had experienced the sensation of a strong contraction produced by electrical stimulation. It is unlikely to cause harm, in any case, and it may help.

## Surgery

It is tempting to imagine, since we believe that stress incontinence is usually caused by a flaw in the anatomy of the system, that modern surgical techniques could correct the fault in a single operation, permanently, completely, with little risk and no further effort. Sadly, surgery is not such a perfect treatment.

Some damage is inevitable in any operation because the surgeon has to cut through healthy tissues and, although they heal, they scar. It is worthwhile when the good outweighs the harm. If there is a distinct, repairable injury or deformity (such as a fistula), the benefits are far greater than the costs and in these situations surgery is the most, or even the only, appropriate treatment. However, in most cases of stress incontinence the defect is more subtle and the balance between good and harm is more delicate.

There are various operations in use. Some are meant to narrow the gap between the pelvic floor muscles while others are intended to give more solid support under the bladder neck. Some place a sling under the urethra to hold it in the abdominal cavity. The approach may be through the wall of the vagina or through the abdomen; many surgeons believe that the latter route is more effective. Most reports (e.g. 13, 15, 23) claim a success rate between 70 per cent and 90 per cent, although for some procedures[12,18] it is below 50 per cent. The degree of success depends on the selection of the patients, the choice of procedure and the length of time since the operation, declining as time passes.

There are some doctors who still believe that surgery is the only effective treatment for incontinence but in most cases it should not be the first choice. It is much more sensible to try the 'conservative' approaches first and resort to surgery only when necessary, which will only be occasionally. An unsuccessful operation is worse than useless because it leaves scars which make it more difficult (though still not impossible) to achieve a good result by exercise or by a second operation. On the other hand, the gentler treatments do not affect surgery adversely. In fact, most surgeons nowadays would advise you to exercise before and after an operation as the better the condition of your pelvic floor muscles, the better the result is likely to be.

Before deciding on surgery, your problem should be very carefully investigated in order to work out which operation, if any, has the best chance of success. In some cases, for example if the incontinence is caused by bladder instability, no operation directed at the supporting structures will help. Hysterectomies and operations to correct prolapse of the uterus or vagina are not even designed to improve incontinence so take them only if they are required for their own purposes.

A well-chosen operation will probably (but not certainly) improve or even cure your symptoms. To weigh against that potential benefit you need to know something of the risks. The use of a general anaesthetic carries some risk in itself, which is why surgery is not offered unless you are in reasonable physical condition, and there is always the possibility of infection in the wound. However good and careful the surgeon, there is also a chance of accidental injury, over and above a degree of unavoidable damage, and this could actually make your symptoms worse. Some operations have recognized discomforts attached. For example, you might have to use a catheter for several weeks before bladder emptying returned to normal after a sling operation, and bladder instability sometimes develops after other types of operation.

If you are considering surgery, talk to the doctors very carefully. They should be prepared to explain exactly what they are proposing to do and why they think it will help in your particular case. They should also be able to tell you what are the chances of your being cured, improved or unchanged, what complications are possible and how likely they are. Take as much time as you need for thinking before you decide. Surgery can be highly effective but it is not reversible and not free of risk, so it is right to be cautious. It is not usually offered until your family is complete in case injury is repeated in a subsequent pregnancy or birth.

## Teflon Injection

In this method, an inert paste of teflon is injected around the urethra with the idea of increasing its resistance to urine flow. It may appear a less drastic technique than surgery but it is no more reversible, no more reliable and rather less precise. Not recommended.

## Drugs

When hormone loss (usually following the menopause) is contributing to the bladder problem, hormone replacement can be useful, but stress incontinence in general is not very amenable to drug treatment. All the available drugs have side-effects because they influence the muscles of the bladder or urethra indirectly by acting on nerves, and of course they act on nerves affecting other parts of the body too. They are helpful in some selected cases but they are not a simple cure-all.

## Mechanical aids

Various mechanical devices have been devised and discarded over the years. They were worn in, or partly in, the vagina and were intended to close the urethra or to support the bladder neck. Each version was useful in some cases but none was altogether satisfactory. However, even if a mechanical device is not very good, it has one huge advantage over surgical treatments for incontinence: if you do not get on with it, you can take it out and perhaps try another one. If you have not been successful with other treatments and are unwilling or unsuitable for surgery, do ask whether any mechanical aids are available. You may be lucky enough to find one that suits you.

# Some questions answered

**Is it worth trying to cure my stress incontinence when I am planning to have another baby? Surely I will just land back where I started after the birth.**

Yes, it is worth it even though the next baby will set you back a bit. If you ignore the problem now, and go into the pregnancy with weak pelvic floor muscles, by the time they have been damaged by another cycle of childbearing you will not just be back where you started but even worse off. If you are to recover as quickly and completely as possible you must get the muscles into good shape now and be ready to start exercising them again immediately after the birth.

If you are pregnant already, it is a real effort to keep going with the exercise because, until the baby is born, you can do little more than prevent the incontinence worsening but it is still worthwhile because it will enable you to make speedy progress after the birth.

Stress incontinence during pregnancy is very common but do not accept it as just another of those inconvenient side effects like swollen ankles which will pass when the pregnancy ends. It is a clear signal of weakness in the mechanism for closing the urethra and you should start doing something about it straight away.

## What about other exercises? Do they help or might they make things worse?

General exercise has such important benefits for your health, both short-term and long-term, that you certainly want to keep it up in some form. It would not be a good bargain to exchange incontinence for the illness of unfitness.

There is very little evidence to show an effect of general exercise on incontinence one way or the other although at least one group has noticed that weakening of the abdominal muscles is often linked with the recurrence of incontinence.[23] In two small studies,[20,21] additional exercises, such as flattening the lower back against the floor and squeezing a cushion between the knees, were prescribed along with pelvic floor exercise, all to be done with the pelvic floor held tight. It is not clear whether the extra exercises made much difference to the cure of incontinence but no doubt they improved the condition of the other muscles involved, and the results were no worse than in other studies.

Gordon and Logue[6] found that about a year after having their babies the women who had done postnatal exercises, and especially those who had continued to take regular exercise, had stronger pelvic muscles than the others. They therefore felt that general exercise strengthened the pelvic floor but this small study was not conclusive. Perhaps the women with weaker pelvic muscles suffered more from incontinence and so were put off from exercising, rather than developing pelvic muscle weakness as a result of a slothful lifestyle.

Jolleys[8] noticed that incontinence was commoner amongst women who did pelvic floor exercise but she did not suppose that the exercise caused the incontinence. It is more probably the other way round; the women with stress incontinence choose to do the exercises because they feel they need to, while those with good bladder control give them up.

As a general rule, it is not helpful to overstrain or overstretch any muscle so if you can feel that the exercise you do puts a strain on your pelvic floor, it could be slowing your recovery. Consider having a break from those particular exercises for a few weeks or months while you build up your pelvic muscle strength. At the very least, pull up your pelvic floor while you do exercises like situps or lifting weights which put pressure on it.

Another piece of practical advice is not to do the pelvic floor exercises immediately before your run or aerobics class. The pelvic muscles would be fatigued and so less able to prevent leaks during your exercise session.

There is no question that leaking urine while you exercise takes away a lot of the enjoyment and satisfaction. One obvious strategy is to change to an activity which keeps you fit without causing leaks, perhaps swimming or cycling instead of running or aerobics. Another strategy is to use the most effective absorbent pads you can buy and carry on with your old sport. Whichever you choose, remember that you have only managed your problem, not cured it completely. You may not leak (because you do not run), or you may be able to do all the things you want (because you wear pads), but to solve the problem at root you still need to work at your pelvic floor exercises.

## Can the pelvic floor exercises cause any harm?

It is hard to think of any injury you could possibly cause simply by using your pelvic floor muscles. The only reported side-effect, as with other exercise programs, is mild muscle ache in the first week or two. It is just possible to imagine side-effects from the stop stream exercise, though none has been documented, so it is sensible to give that up once it has served its purpose i.e. when you can do it or when symptoms lessen.

## What about sex? Is it likely to make my incontinence worse?

No. A penis will not stretch the pelvic floor muscles excessively; the normal gap between them is quite wide enough for intercourse. If anything, sex should help because it makes the muscles contract automatically and so exercises them.

# Summing Up

- practise holding on to your urine and stopping the stream.
- do pelvic lifts, holding for five seconds and relaxing for five seconds, in sets of six lifts, ten to thirty sets per day.
- keep records and keep going!

# Chapter 8

# FREQUENCY, URGENCY AND RELATED PROBLEMS

Bladder training is a method of gradually increasing the time between your visits to the toilet so that, by degrees, your bladder becomes able to hold larger quantities of urine comfortably. It is a highly effective treatment for 'primary' urge incontinence, urgency and frequency (i.e. where the symptoms are not secondary to some separate disorder) and it is also useful against bedwetting and nocturia.

It is not suitable for urgency and frequency caused by cystitis, nor for symptoms caused by obstruction of the urethra. If you have cystitis due to an infection, trying to overcome it with bladder training is sure to make it worse. The proper treatment for cystitis is explained in Chapter 11. If you have longstanding symptoms that you want to treat with bladder training but also have some suspicion that you may have a bladder infection, you must be sure that the infection is cleared up before you start the training schedule. See your doctor and explain the situation; a simple test on a urine sample is enough to check whether there are bacteria infecting it or not.

Read Chapter 3 if you have any other symptoms and are uncertain about whether or not you should consult your doctor.

## Bladder Training — What to Do

By the time you reach this point in the book, you should have read Chapter 6 and have a record of your bladder's behaviour at the moment. If not, go back and observe your bladder emptying pattern for a few days. You need to know how long you go between deliberate emptyings, what volume you produce and how often you lose urine accidentally, and you need to know all this before you start the training program so that you will be able to see your progress.

Now look at your record of urine volumes and see what your highest reading was. Your bladder is physically capable of holding at least that amount of urine every time but probably most of the readings were well below the maximum. A common pattern is to feel a need to produce small amounts of urine very often during the day, but to have a full night's sleep and produce 300 ml (10 fluid ounces) or more in the morning. A bladder can be remarkably convincing in insisting that it needs emptying when it is really only part full, particularly when you are awake!

There is nothing complicated in the idea of bladder training. You just have to hang on for longer between trips to the loo until you can last four hours comfortably and confidently. It is certainly very hard work at first but you can make quite a lot of progress in a week or two which will help motivate you to carry on.

There are two approaches to increasing the time between emptyings. One is to wait for the urge, then delay going for a few minutes and gradually increase the delay between urge and emptying. When you learn to overcome an urge so completely that it actually passes away, you go on to repeat the delaying tactics with the next urge. This works very well if you are tenacious enough. You do have to decide when you have done enough delaying, though — whether to hang on for ten minutes after this urge, for example, or wait for the next one — and this uncertainty can dilute your determination.

The other approach is to set a fixed time between loo trips for the day and overcome all urges which occur before the scheduled time. This works very well too if you are resolute and, because it is more definite, there are fewer decisions and it is more difficult to cheat yourself. This method is probably the better one unless your symptoms are relatively mild.

# Choosing the Interval

If you have decided to use the delay-after-urge method, start with a two-minute delay. After a day or two, increase the delay to five minutes and so long as you are successful with it, add an extra five minutes each day until you are holding on for half an hour. If the urge is disappearing before the time is up, wait for it to re-appear before you go to the toilet, and gradually postpone the trip after this second urge as well. If you find that the urge does not disappear, just increase the delay steadily until you are lasting four hours or producing 400 ml (14 fluid ounces) of urine in one go.

If you have chosen the fixed-interval method, have a look at your urinary diary and see what was your longest interval during the day. Start with an interval similar to that; an hour and a half is about right for most people but there is no harm in starting lower and working up. Each day that you are successful, increase the interval for the next day by ten minutes. You can reach the target of four hours in a fortnight, though it will take longer before your new voiding pattern becomes an effortless habit.

# Overcoming the Urge

Once you have chosen your interval, you must regard it as absolute. Insist to yourself that you simply will not go into the toilet until the time is up, whatever the consequences. You can think of it as a straight fight for control between you and your bladder. It is a fight that you can win, but in the past your bladder has been in the habit of bossing you rather than the other way about so you need to make it perfectly clear that you mean business. When you say that there will be an hour and a half between voids, you must mean it!

The most important thing to know is that most of the times when your bladder signals that it is full, it is lying to you and does not actually need to be emptied. Remember: whatever the highest volume on your record was, your bladder can already hold at least that much. Tell yourself very firmly that you do not need to go or, if you find that anger helps, swear at your low-down mendacious deceitful bladder and promise that you won't be taken in this time.

BLADDER PROBLEMS

Then use every trick in the book to hold on to your urine until the urge passes off and you can release it at your own chosen time.

Pull up your pelvic floor muscles as strongly as you can without tensing your tummy and hold them tight. If you are not sure about your pelvic floor muscles, have a look at Chapter 7 for some hints on learning to make them work for you. As well as helping to compress the urethra and prevent urine leakage directly, there is a reflex pathway which tends to make the bladder muscle relax when the pelvic floor is contracted.

Put pressure upwards between your legs, more towards the front than the back. Experiment to find the spot that works best for you. This not only helps to prevent a leak but actually helps to relieve the voiding urge. If you are alone, you can just hold yourself with a hand. Otherwise cross your legs, sit on the arm of a chair, crouch down so that you sit on the heel of one foot or do anything else that helps you to keep control of your bladder. Obviously, you will want to do away with these manoeuvres eventually but to begin with the priority is simply to make it through your allotted time without leaking.

You will probably find it easier to hold on if you lean forward or sit rather than standing. Once you are in a good position to resist the urge, don't move until you feel that you are back in control.

Thinking of emptying your bladder is the most unhelpful thing you can do now, so you need to banish all thoughts of toilets by filling your mind with something else. It does not matter what you use as the alternative so long as you really concentrate on it. If you already have some good method of distracting yourself, use that. Breathing relaxation is very good if you have practised it — deep, slow, regular breaths, concentrating on nothing but the air moving slowly in and out of your lungs. Otherwise, try any of the following:

- mental arithmetic — work out how many pints of milk you use in a year, or how many letters there are in the first verse of the national anthem.

- reciting poetry — if you can get all the way through 'The Rime of the Ancient Mariner' you deserve a medal for your memory as well as for your bladder control.

- imagery — retrace some familiar journey in your mind, filling in all the details as you go along.
- something useful — work out next week's shopping list or compose a letter to a friend.

Once you have managed the first peak of the urge to empty your bladder you can start moving about and getting on with whatever you were doing before. It may be sensible, particularly in the early stages, to avoid activities which you know tend to provoke your bladder. For instance, washing up and anything which involves the sploshing of water is liable to suggest a need to urinate (this is not an old wives' tale, there is good evidence for it![15]), so these are jobs to do soon after you have emptied your bladder, not when you have just staved off an attack of urgency. Concentrate on what you are doing or carry on using the distraction techniques to keep your mind busy on something other than your bladder.

Even if you are due for a toilet trip when you notice that your bladder is signalling a need to void, do not rush off until you have the urge under control. Hurrying makes it all the more difficult to prevent a leak. Stop and use the usual tricks to hold sway over your bladder, then set off cautiously so that the movement does not set the urge off again. Stop on the way as well if need be.

# Keeping Records

Keeping a record of the intervals between voidings is an essential part of the method so make sure that you have a small notebook always handy. Whenever you empty your bladder deliberately, make a note of the time. Do it then, do not leave it and try to remember later. Also keep a note of all the times you successfully overcome an urge to void, and all the times you leak.

It is not necessary to measure the volume every time. Of course you can if you like, but it is not very practicable if you are out and about and it can be demoralizing if you have valiantly hung on for two hours to find that the amount of urine in your bladder was well below your personal best. It is enough to measure volumes just one day a week as you did when your were sizing up the problem before you started the training program.

You will see your progress in the increasing intervals between your visits to the toilet and in the number of times you succeed in resisting the urge to empty your bladder. You will also see progress as the volume of urine you produce each time increases and approaches your original maximum volume. Your maximum volume will increase too; eventually it should reach the normal level of 400 ml (14 fluid ounces) or more.

Do not be downcast if you seem to have more leaks than before in the early days of the training program. It is a passing stage where you are no longer pre-empting leaks by voiding every half hour but have not yet retrained your bladder to accept the longer intervals uncomplainingly. Stick steadfastly to the new regime and you can achieve both advantages together — longer intervals and fewer leaks.

# Sticking to the Program

The first few days of the bladder training program will be hard going. Expect to succeed, but do not expect it to be easy. After you have successfully beaten off the first few urges to empty your bladder, it is natural to feel that you have proved your point and that your bladder should cease its unreasonable demands. It won't. It will throw up many more misleading desires to void, and you will have to deal with every last one of them. Of course, on the later occasions, you will have the advantage of knowing that you can resist the urge because you have done it before, but still you will wish sometimes that there was no need for resistance. Just remember what you stand to gain. It must be worth the effort of tackling even the umpteenth urge of the evening when you have the chance of banishing your bladder problem permanently.

At night you can relax your vigilance. During the day, as instructor to a delinquent bladder, you cannot let any misbehaviour pass uncontested, but once you get to bed you are off-duty. Even if you have night-time symptoms to overcome, do not try to continue the bladder drill beyond bedtime. You need your sleep more than your bladder needs the extra training. If you are woken by a bladder claiming to be full, just empty it and go back to sleep. As you make progress with your daytime training program, the need to void at night will naturally fade away.

To give yourself the best chance of success, try to start your program at a time that gives you a clear week, or better still a fortnight, to concentrate on it. It is discouraging to start at a weekend, make some small progress, and then find it impossible to hold to your schedule on Monday because your work requires you to be in certain places at certain times. Apart from the demands of the occupation itself, it is hard to stick to your new regime if your colleagues all expect you to behave in your old way.

Early on, when bladder training was a new idea, a woman would be taken into hospital for the first week or two in order to remove her from these pressures, but this is done less often now. Doctors found that the success rate was equally high if they treated the women as outpatients and the inpatient treatment was expensive as well as being disruptive to the woman and her family. Still, if you would have liked a doctor to prescribe you a week in hospital to start sorting out your bladder problem, perhaps you can prescribe yourself a week's holiday for the job.

Arrange to be busy on some sort of project that will keep you occupied without making you anxious, painting the living room for instance. It is easier to ignore the desire to empty your bladder if you have something else to get on with. It also provides an innocuous answer in case you want one for workmates who ask what you will be doing in your week off. It is for you to choose whom to tell about your bladder training regime, and when, and you may well choose not to tell these people at this time. You might possibly manage the whole program without telling anybody at work at any time, but I would not advocate such a degree of secrecy. It will be easier if you take your close colleagues into your confidence so that they can support you and discourage backsliding when you return to the old routine.

Whoever will be your companions during the first week or so, recruit them to your cause if you possibly can. If they can give you positive moral support, so much the better. At least, if you tell them what you are trying to do, they should have the consideration not to demand that you break your schedule to fit in with their convenience. If they are going to undermine your efforts, no matter how nicely or humorously, think very hard how to have some time apart. Visit a relative, have a week in a holiday cottage, send the family on an expedition to the North Pole. Just for once, be quite selfish about it. If your bladder problem is wrecking your life, a week on your own to get to grips with it is not too much to ask. The family can fend for themselves for that long, just as they would have to if you spent the week in hospital, and they will share the benefits when you have done all the hard work of bladder training and got the problem under control.

Do not feel that it is impossible to retrain your bladder if you cannot get time away from your usual duties. It takes more planning to reconcile the demands of your bladder training with the demands of your occupation, and it takes longer to reach your goals if you cannot stick to the program throughout the day, but it can be done. A clear week to start the schedule is a great help, but you can succeed without if need be. Keep up the recording of all your deliberate urinations and all your leaks without a break even if there are periods when you cannot follow the active training regime.

Whether or not you manage to shed most of your normal responsibilities, it will be all too easy to find excuses to duck your time targets. Watch out for the temptations and resist them. 'Oh, I must just go to the loo even though it's only an hour since last time because I have to go to the shops . . .' Nonsense. Wait to empty your bladder on schedule, then shop. Or, at the proper time, use the toilet in the shopping centre. Your training program is your number one priority for now so plan your other activities around it, and never mind if you have to miss some things out for a couple of weeks. Once you have your problem on the run (instead of the other way about) you will be able to take up all your old pastimes and some more besides.

Another way of cheating yourself is by reducing the amount you drink. This may make it possible to hold on longer but it certainly will not help you to teach your bladder to hold a normal amount of urine. In fact, concentrated urine seems to encourage the desire to void more than dilute urine does, so it may even make it harder to get through your allotted times. Drink plenty, and spread it evenly through the day to avoid sudden surges in urine production. A steady inflow is less likely to provoke your bladder into signalling a spurious need to be emptied.

Avoid pads as much as possible, certainly while you are on your own at home. Obviously you care about leaking whether or not you are wearing a pad, but being pad-free gives your efforts to overcome unwelcome urges an extra degree of importance. It also helps you to be aware of exactly how successful you have been. As your success grows, your confidence can grow with it.

Bladder training is different from pelvic floor exercise because you see the first signs of progress much sooner. Within a week, you will have won the first skirmish, overcome some urges and held out longer between visits to the toilet. Encouraged by that success, it is not too difficult to motivate yourself to carry on. Later on, there may be times when progress seems to have stopped, perhaps when you are able to hold urine for several hours at a stretch but are still bothered by many unnecessary urges to release it. Be stubborn! Keep going! Eventually the urges will get weaker too but it does take time.

Until your new habits are very well established, be quite deliberate about sticking to them. Do not let some small venture such as a car journey start you back into the old way of frequent bladder emptying. You know that you can manage a certain time between voids, it makes no difference whether you are in a car or in your own home, and you certainly need not visit the lavatory 'just in case'. In case of what? You can always find somewhere to empty your bladder. If the place is inhabited, there are toilets and you can ask to use one; if it is uninhabited there will be no-one to see you 'behind a bush'. It would be ironic, when the point of the training was to enable you to undertake such enterprises in comfort, if you let the thought of one undo all your good work.

# Reviewing Progress

After three months, stop and see how you are getting on. There is a fair chance that you will be without symptoms and quite happy with the result. Tremendous! Now you can recommend the treatment to all your friends who are still emptying their bladders on the 'never miss a chance' system.

A likelier possibility is that you will be very much improved but still have some way to go before you could call your bladder control perfect. If so, carry on with the training program. You can expect your remaining symptoms to diminish gradually as your bladder becomes more accustomed to holding larger volumes of urine for longer periods of time.

If you feel that you are no better, first check your most recent bladder record against your original one. You may find that you have made some progress after all and, even though you have not reached your goal yet, you should be encouraged enough to take up training again with renewed determination. If you have really made no progress, consider how earnestly you followed the schedule. It is a very obvious point that bladder training only works if you actually do it, and failing to do it is the commonest reason for failing to succeed. If that was your problem, tear up any records you did make, go back to Chapter 6 and start all over again. If you are sure that you followed the training diligently and have had no benefit, consult a doctor.

You may find that, although you have overcome most or all of your bladder problem, you are still nervous about taking up normal activities again. This is understandable, especially if you had had the problem for a long time and lost a lot of confidence, but all your work in bladder training will have been rather wasted unless you make the effort to get over this last hurdle. Approach it in the same way that you approached the original training program. Start with short outings and work up gradually but deliberately. Remember, there is no reason to expect any difficulty. If you can hold urine for hours at a stretch at home, you can do the same wherever you are.

When you are satisfied with the state you have reached, you obviously need not keep to the rigid pattern of the training schedule. Do still be on your guard against drifting back into the old habit of frequent bladder emptying, though. Make a habit of charting your bladder's behaviour at intervals, say one day a month. Then you will notice very early if you are tending to visit the toilet more often, or having to hurry to reach it, and a short period of deliberate bladder training will be enough to put you back on course.

# Will it Work?

70-90 per cent of the women who reach specialist clinics and are treated by bladder drill are cured or much improved three months after the start of the treatment. This picture is consistent across a number of studies by at least seven separate research teams.[2,3,5,6,8,9,10,14,16] Assuming that, like the large majority of women who share your problem, you have no serious illness at the root of your difficulty, your chances should be at least as good.

The do-it-yourself regime is basically the same as the bladder training used in these studies but there are some differences between the two situations. You will not go to hospital, for instance, nor will you take medicines intended to pacify your bladder. Most of the women in the research projects spent some time in hospital and most were given drugs, at least initially, but it probably made little difference to the final result. The patients treated by Pengelly and Booth[14] received no drugs but still three quarters of them were improved or cured and it made no difference whether they stayed in hospital or went as out-patients. Frewen's patients achieved an excellent success rate with neither drugs nor a hospital stay;[6] 78 out of 90 were completely symptom-free after three months and all but two had improved.

Another difference is that you will be relying on your own resources rather than the support and encouragement of medical staff. No doubt encouragement is helpful, hence the importance of enlisting the support of your family and friends if possible. Expert supportive counselling may even have some effect on its own.[11] But, in the end, what really matters is to complete the course. Thus, of the women who failed to benefit in Millard & Oldenburg's clinic, over half had failed to complete the three months' training.[13] Macaulay's team[11] found that women taught bladder drill in an intentionally non-empathetic, non-supportive way gained little ground but this is hardly surprising. How much effort would you put into a bladder training program presented with such a calculated lack of enthusiasm?

You have already shown that you have more than the usual degree of independence and determination simply by the fact that you are planning to take on the problem yourself. You therefore have an excellent chance of sticking to the schedule for three months, and if you do that you have an excellent chance of success.

There is one more difference between you and the women in the research studies which should encourage you. They had very severe symptoms, severe enough to drive them to their doctors who then referred them to specialists; some of them had already tried other treatments without success. Even so, the large majority were successful with bladder training. If your symptoms are somewhat milder, which is likely, the outlook is that much brighter still.

## How long will it take?

There will be a noticeable change in two weeks [14] and you can learn to hold urine for three to four hours in less than three weeks. [10] After three months roughly four out of five women are at least substantially improved. The number totally cured by this time varies in different reports from about 30 per cent upwards. With further training there is further progress, so women who are prepared to stick with the scheme beyond three months are very likely to achieve complete success in the end.

Frewen [6] found that waking to empty the bladder at night was usually the first symptom to go. He also warned that, even after frequency and incontinence were under control, it would be several months before unstable bladders would become stable and urgency no longer a problem.

Mahady and Begg [12] used a rather gentler scheme of training, concentrating on keeping bladder record charts and not making any special effort to delay urination. They found that it took an average of five months after overcoming actual incontinence before the last of the other symptoms disappeared. In this study, 75 per cent of the women were dry by 6 months and the number continued to rise, reaching 85 per cent by 12 months and 90 per cent by 18 months. About 40 per cent were rid of all their symptoms within 6 months. This figure also rose as the women continued with the program, 65 per cent being symptom-free after a year and 85 per cent after two years.

Once you have beaten your bladder problem, be vigilant to prevent it recurring. In one report,[8] almost half the women whose symptoms had improved on a three-month bladder training program relapsed in the following one to five years. It is not obvious why so many of this group fell by the wayside as the cure can be long lasting. All of the women cured in Mahady and Begg's study remained cured 4 years after starting the treatment[12] and Frewen too found that a very high proportion of the women he had treated were still well six years later.[7] So long as you are watchful and tackle minor lapses before they have a chance to become re-established as habits, you can expect your cure to be permanent.

# Alternatives
## Hypnotherapy

Freeman and Baxby treated fifty women with twelve sessions of hypnotherapy over a month.[4] Forty-three of them were improved or cured, a success rate very similar to that obtained by bladder training alone. In fact the women also kept urinary diaries throughout the treatment period so they were using a form of bladder training in addition to the hypnosis.

Using hypnosis probably adds little to do-it-yourself bladder training but, in the hands of a competent therapist, it is unlikely to do you any harm, and you may find it helpful. Some conventional doctors are also trained in hypnotherapy. Other therapists are not medically qualified but have earned membership of the British Hypnotherapy Society while others again have no qualifications at all.

## Drugs

Medicines are available (on doctor's prescription only) which reduce bladder activity and these can be helpful if your symptoms are related to detrusor instability. They act on the nerve pathways which control the bladder and as there are similar nerves in other parts of the body, side effects are common. They are not generally recommended for long-term use. These drugs can be useful in a bladder training program as they help you to achieve early and encouraging success, but then you need to wean yourself off them and learn to rely on your own control. They are not a complete answer in themselves.

# Biofeedback

Biofeedback is intended to help patients learn to control their bladder muscle by displaying its behaviour moment by moment. The success rate is no higher than that of ordinary bladder training.[1] It requires sophisticated equipment for the simultaneous measurement of pressures inside the bladder and vagina, and it is immensely time-consuming for both the patients and the medical staff. It is not a popular technique and it is available only by referral to specialist centres.

# Surgery

If the underlying cause of the symptoms is obstruction of the urethra, surgery is an appropriate and effective treatment. Once the blockage is removed the bladder has a chance to return to more normal behaviour. However, if there is no obvious reason for your bladder's unstable behaviour the outlook for surgical treatment is much less encouraging.

It is quite possible to perform operations which reduce the efficiency of unwanted bladder contractions by interrupting the nerve networks in the bladder wall. These operations reduce urge incontinence but they have a major drawback as they also diminish the efficiency of normal emptying contractions. This makes it likely that urine would be left in the bladder, giving a real risk of urinary infections, and you might need to use techniques like abdominal pressure to help empty your bladder. You might even have to use a catheter at regular intervals to release the urine.

In some cases urge incontinence is so intensely distressing that surgery is worthwhile, but it is not an easy option and there is no going back so you would need to discuss it very carefully before you made your choice.

# Phenol

Phenol is the chemical which used to give hospitals their characteristic carbolic disinfectant smell. It damages nerves and it can be used to disrupt the nerve pathways which co-ordinate contractions of the bladder muscle.

The technique of treatment with phenol is simpler than surgery but the result is similar. Unwanted contractions may be reduced or abolished but so is the normal activity of the bladder. It therefore has considerable disadvantages, just as surgery has, and the effects are permanent.

# Chapter 9

# BEDWETTING

To have an unbroken and dry night's sleep, your bladder needs to be able to hold all the urine produced between bedtime and morning. If it cannot hold a whole night's output but you wake when it is full, you will suffer from nocturia; your sleep will be disturbed but you will keep a dry bed. You will only suffer from bedwetting if your full bladder fails to wake you up.

We do not know why some people wake easily when their bladders are full while others carry on sleeping. It could be that the signals coming from their bladders are weaker than normal, or it could be that they sleep unusually heavily.

There is not a great deal you can do to make yourself sleep more lightly. Caffeine (in drinks like coffee) is definitely not recommended as it actually increases the production of urine. It would probably not be effective in any case; even very strong stimulants like amphetamine which doctors sometimes used in the past were not hugely successful in reducing bedwetting.

However, it is possible to eliminate those things which make you sleep more heavily — alcohol in the evenings, for instance. If you take sleeping pills, consult your doctor about giving them up. In fact it is worth talking to your doctor about the problem if you are taking any medicines at all, as all sorts of drugs may have the side-effect of making you sleepy. Some drugs can also increase the production of urine or interfere with the mechanism which normally slows down urine production at night and these too could make your problem worse.

The only other approach to your sleepfulness is an alarm clock. This is not a cure by any means, but as a purely practical measure you might well prefer a broken night to a wet bed. If you normally wake up after wetting the bed you will have some idea of the time when the enuresis usually happens and you can set the clock to wake you shortly beforehand. Otherwise you will have to find the best time for the alarm call by trial and error; you can gain a clue as to the likely interval by seeing how long you can go between voids during the day. If you find that you can successfully pre-empt your leaks like this, why not try very gradually setting the clock for longer intervals?

The alarm clock idea is simple but it does have some drawbacks. One is that, if you only have accidents occasionally, you will often be waking yourself unnecessarily. Another point is that you are developing a habit of emptying your bladder during the night, a habit which could conceivably make bedwetting more likely if you stop using the clock. Finally, unless you try sleeping some nights without the clock, you will never know when you stop needing it. I suggest that you try the other self-help ideas in this chapter first without waking yourself, but keep the possibility of using an alarm clock in mind as a practical strategy for special occasions.

Sleeping through the signals from your full bladder is only one half of your problem; the other half is that your bladder becomes full in the first place. There are two possible reasons for this. It may be that your bladder holds less urine than most, or it may be that you produce more urine during the night than other people.

You can get a good idea of the working capacity of your bladder by measuring the volume of urine every time you empty it, as explained in Chapter 6. If you always void much less than 400ml (14 fluid ounces), or can only reach 400ml by holding on much longer than is comfortable, then your bladder does not have the capacity to hold a normal night's output of urine easily. You probably have frequency as well as bedwetting, and perhaps urgency or urge incontinence as well. You need to train your bladder to hold larger amounts of liquid by following the program in Chapter 8.

Follow the bladder training schedule until you can hold your urine comfortably for four hours and produce 400ml with reasonable ease. Your bedwetting may cease promptly when you can hold 400ml but do not be surprised if it persists until you have kept up your new voiding pattern for several weeks. If your bladder was unstable to begin with, as it is in about 75 per cent of people with enuresis,[1,3,6] it will take some time after you have established a normal daytime voiding pattern before the unstable contractions cease. When you are asleep, you cannot deliberately resist your bladder's attempts to empty itself, as you can when you are awake, so you should not expect the bedwetting to stop until your bladder has had plenty of practice in holding the required amount of liquid.

Your chances of success with the bladder training treatment are high. Of 26 women treated with bladder drill by Jarvis,[4] 17 were completely cured and two more improved. The cure lasted at least as long as the follow-up period (6 to 14 months) even though the initial training program itself had been short (5 to 16 days).

As well as aiming to increase the capacity of your bladder, it is worth taking simple steps to reduce the amount of urine produced overnight. This does not mean depriving yourself of drinks from mid-afternoon onwards. As I explained in Chapter 6, it is not helpful to try to reduce your fluid intake drastically in the attempt to overcome any form of incontinence. All the same, you should think again about those couple of quick ones just before the bar closes; they are bound to reach the other end of your system during the night and increase your chances of waking in a wet bed. Alcoholic 'shorts' are no better than long drinks in this respect as they make you produce a volume of urine much larger than the original drink. If you have not drunk extra water, your kidneys will simply take what they need from other parts of your body. You may feel dehydrated and dreadful in the morning but your bladder will certainly have filled — and perhaps emptied — during the night.

As a general guide, drink plenty during the day (3 pints or more) but reduce your fluid intake and cut out caffeinated drinks completely in the three or four hours before bedtime.

Caffeine remains active in the body for several hours so, if you are taking in large amounts during the day, four hours without coffee in the evening may not be long enough for it to be cleared from your system before you go to bed. You could well benefit more by banishing caffeine from your diet altogether. Edelstein[2] reported a study in which he replaced all caffeinated drinks in a large psychiatric hospital with decaffeinated substitutes. The main area of interest was not enuresis but eight of the residents in the study had previously wet their beds at least three times a week and they all, quite unexpectedly, showed a marked reduction in the number of wet nights when caffeine was withdrawn.

There is no real way of knowing whether the root cause of your difficulty is a small effective bladder capacity, a large overnight urine production, or an unusual sleep pattern, so the best way forward is to take action against all three possibilities. Use bladder training to enlarge your bladder capacity; avoid caffeine and regulate your intake of fluid in the evening to avoid excessive urine production; cut out alcohol in the evening, and consult your doctor about medicines which may be affecting your sleep or your urine output. When the bedwetting stops you can try re-introducing the things you have missed. Restart them one at a time so that if your problem recurs you will know what it was that probably caused the relapse.

Keep a careful record of every night you stay dry so that you can see your progress. Ignore the wet nights as much as you can. Of course it is disappointing to have a wet night when you have had a few dry ones and were beginning to hope that you had your problem completely beaten, but reaching your goal is bound to be a gradual process. It is much more helpful to concentrate on the fact that you have gone up from, say, one night dry in the week to four and realize that your self-help program is working than to think that because you are still wet sometimes you are not getting anywhere.

After three months of determined effort on the bladder training program you can expect to see substantial progress. You may have reached a point where you are happy with your bladder control, or you may want to carry on for another few months to improve even more. However, if you have followed the program honestly, and honestly feel that you are very little better than you were three months ago, do consult a doctor.

# Alternatives

Any of the treatments described in Chapter 8 for urgency and related symptoms might be considered for bedwetting but there are two additional treatments which are designed especially for it.

## Drugs

Desmopressin is a synthetic version of a hormone normally produced in your brain. The natural hormone is called vasopressin or anti-diuretic hormone and it reduces the volume of urine you produce. Your brain produces more vasopressin when you are short of water and most people also produce more of it at night. Some people with enuresis apparently do not produce extra vasopressin at night [5] and they may be helped by taking a small dose of the synthetic version late in the evening to reduce their urine output overnight.

## Pad-and-bell Bladder Training

This involves a sensitive pad in your bed, pants or pyjama trousers which will sound a bell or buzzer to wake you up as soon as urine escapes. With luck, you will be able to stop the flow and complete the process at the toilet.

The idea of the treatment is that you get so used to waking with a full bladder that, after a while, you will wake automatically without the need for a bell and before the bed gets wet. It is quite a good method and worth trying even if you have used something similar in the past without success. Your bladder control system has probably matured since then and other circumstances (such as where you live, and with whom) may have changed too.

Of all the bladder problems, bedwetting is possibly one of the hardest to admit to. The stereotype of the bedwetter as a child, smelly, outcast and unhappy at school, is a powerful image which lingers like a spectre to undermine your confidence in yourself and your trust in others. With the help of the methods described here, and possibly a doctor's advice as well, you can hope to set the ghost to rest for good.

# Chapter 10

# IN COMPANY
## — GIGGLE INCONTINENCE AND INCONTINENCE DURING INTERCOURSE

## Giggle Incontinence

Probably the worst thing about giggle incontinence is that it so often happens in company, simply because the funniest things always do seem to happen when you are with your friends. It is annoying enough to wet yourself in private but it can be acutely embarrassing, humiliating even, when other people are there.

Giggle incontinence is quite common in young children and usually cures itself without anybody doing anything about it. If a four-year-old wets her pants over a good joke and nobody makes a big fuss, the child herself does not feel excessively ashamed and she does not worry that the same thing may happen again. In time the accidents just stop happening. The situation is different — and much more problematical — if laughter still causes leaks when you are old enough to be upset and worried by them. Then the fear of having an accident not only spoils your enjoyment of funny events but actually makes the incontinence more likely to occur.

There are two approaches to the problem of giggle incontinence. The first is at the point where you laugh. In other words, cultivate your serious side and your straight face. This is quite an effective strategy, and there is a natural tendency to become less giggly as you get older anyway, but it is up to you to decide whether you can hurry the process along without losing your personality. You may prefer to be merry but damp rather than dry and humourless.

The second approach, and perhaps the more appealing one, is directly at the point where you leak. There are four useful tips here: posture, pressure, pad and practice.

**Posture:** at the first hint of trouble, sit down. You may be surprised how much easier it is to control your bladder when you are sitting.

**Pressure:** if sitting is not enough, apply pressure to your perineum. A hand between your legs is the most effective but not usually workable in company so sit on the arm of a chair or crouch down so that you are sitting on one heel. The heel-sitting position is good because you can do it anywhere and you can invent good excuses for it, like some form of cramp in your leg. Don't move until the moment has passed and you are back in control of your bladder (see page 94 for more tips on this).

**Pad:** in the early stages, keep your bladder fairly empty while you are with people who make you laugh, and wear a pad. If a leak starts you will be able to stop it quickly by sitting down and applying pressure, and the pad will absorb any small amount of urine that does escape so that there are no telltale damp patches. You will not need the pad for long but it is worth using one in the early stages to relieve anxiety.

**Practice:** practise the stop-flow exercise on page 74. If you find it difficult to stop the flow of urine, practise the pelvic floor exercise on page 75 to strengthen the necessary muscles. If you can stop the flow of urine in mid-stream when you are emptying your bladder deliberately, you will have a better chance of halting any leak produced by laughter.

If you have urgency, frequency or urge incontinence as well as giggle incontinence it may well be that bladder instability is to blame. Read Chapter 6, then go on to the bladder training program in Chapter 8 and you will have a good chance of overcoming it. Bladder training may help you with giggle incontinence even if you are not bothered by other symptoms as it does give extra practice in bladder control.

Following these hints will often deal with the difficulty, and even the passage of time is on your side, so it is seldom necessary to consult a doctor. If you do decide to seek medical help, be prepared for the possibility that your doctor may not be familiar with giggle incontinence as so few sufferers have asked for help in the past. If it is outside your own doctor's area of expertise, and if it is causing you real distress, he may refer you to another doctor who has particular experience or interest in the subject.

# Incontinence During Intercourse

Urine leakage can really spoil sex and contribute to a lot of conflict between a couple but it is not an insoluble problem.

First, take the obvious practical measures to reduce both the scale of the leak and its impact. Empty your bladder before lovemaking; this is good hygiene anyway. Try a different position which puts less pressure on your bladder, particularly if the leak happens on penetration. It is hardly worth protecting the bed against a small leak which only adds a little to the inevitable damp patch, but if leaks are large use a thick towel to save soaking the mattress. Placing it beneath the sheet is more discreet but above is more effective.

Secondly, your incontinence in intercourse is likely to be a symptom either of sphincter weakness (in which case you probably have stress incontinence as well) or of bladder instability (in which case you probably have urgency or frequency or urge incontinence). You will need to deal with these underlying problems by following the treatment in Chapter 7 for suspected sphincter weakness or Chapter 8 for an unstable bladder.

The third thing may be the most difficult to do. If you have not already done so, try to talk it over with your partner. He may be less bothered than you imagine (he has other things on his mind at the time, after all), or he may be more bothered, or he may never have realised how much it bothers you, but until you talk you cannot know how big the problem really is. It may look a lot smaller once you get it out into the open. If talking is very difficult, someone trained in counselling such as a marriage guidance counsellor may be able to help.

# Chapter 11

# CYSTITIS

If you suffer regularly from cystitis you will probably want to read a book dealing with this particular problem in detail; there are several on the market. This chapter gives only the briefest outline, a fire-fighting guide for the first-time sufferer.

## The Symptoms

1. You are likely to have stinging or burning pain when you urinate.

2. You will probably feel that you need to pass urine more often than usual, although the amount of urine you actually produce may be very small.

3. You may feel that you will leak if you do not reach a toilet immediately.

4. You may still want to pass urine when you have only just emptied your bladder.

5. You may feel feverish and have an ache low in your back or abdomen.

6. Your urine may be cloudy or blood-stained.

## Medical Attention

If you are a child, a man or a pregnant woman, see a doctor. Consult a doctor also if you are having repeated attacks of cystitis, if the illness lasts more than a couple of days, or if you are worried by fever, blood in your urine, or any of the other symptoms listed in Chapter 3. While you are waiting for your appointment, follow the self-help routine below.

# Self-Help

Drink loads of water or plain watery drinks — a large mugful every twenty minutes for at least three hours, and a mugful every hour after that. This drinking is the key to the treatment as it washes out bacteria and other irritants from the bladder. Obviously you will need to urinate a lot and this may be painful the first few times but it will get better as the urine becomes more dilute and the inflammation subsides.

There are three other things you can do to make yourself more comfortable but none is so important or effective as the drinking. You can take a teaspoonful of bicarbonate of soda dissolved in a large glass of water once an hour for three hours only (but not if you are pregnant or have heart, kidney, liver or blood pressure problems, or if you are on a low salt diet). It tastes vile but it does help because it makes the urine less acidic so that it stings less and bacteria grow more slowly. Your pharmacist or doctor might be able to tell you of other preparations to try if bicarbonate of soda is unsuitable for you. You can also use a mild painkiller at the dose recommended on the packet and you may find it soothing to put hot water bottles wrapped in towels between your thighs or against your lower back or abdomen.

Your symptoms should begin to wear off after a few hours of this self-help routine, and you should be back to normal in a few days. If not, seek further advice.

# Chapter 12

# HAS YOUR PARTNER GOT A BLADDER PROBLEM?

Actual incontinence is less common in men than in women, but they still have bladder disorders which can cause real distress. You may well be the first to notice the early symptoms of a bladder problem and you could save your partner a good deal of misery if you could persuade him to seek medical advice before they worsen. Symptoms often progress insidiously, and men are just as reluctant as women to approach a doctor for help with a problem so apparently silly as needing to urinate more frequently. Far from being silly, a symptom like this can warn of deeper trouble, or of trouble in the future which might be avoided by timely action.

Men, again like women, may detest the idea of an intimate examination of the problem area, they may feel that 'You have to expect that sort of thing at my age' or they may imagine that there are no suitable treatments. In fact, most bladder problems can be treated and, as with so many medical conditions, treatment is usually both simpler and more effective when given early. It is a mistake to delay seeking help.

## Enlargement of the Prostate Gland

In men, the urethra passes through a gland called the prostate gland which has a role in producing semen and which often becomes enlarged from late middle age onwards. This enlargement is not harmful in itself — hence the medical name for the condition, *benign prostatic hypertrophy* or BPH for short — but of course it squashes the urethra and obstructs urine flow. The situation is made worse by the smooth muscle of the prostate and urethra which tenses up and constricts the urethra even more.

The early symptoms of obstruction of the urethra are hesitancy (i.e. difficulty in starting the flow of urine), a slow stream of urine and an ill-defined dribbling end to urination (terminal dribble). At this stage, a drug which relaxes the tense muscle in the urethra and prostate gland can often relieve the obstruction effectively.

Later, the symptoms of frequency, nocturia and urgency develop and gradually become more severe. It may then be necessary to remove part of the prostate gland surgically. This will usually unblock the urethra and may relieve the symptoms quite promptly. However, if the obstruction has been left untreated for a long time the bladder may well have become unstable. It can revert to stability after the blockage is removed but this does take time and does not always happen; until it does happen the symptoms of frequency and urgency are likely to remain.

# Other Problems

Bedwetting and giggle incontinence affect men in the same way as women and succumb to the same treatments (see Chapters 9 and 10). Any other symptoms should be referred to a doctor.

# GLOSSARY

**ADH:** Antidiuretic hormone, a hormone produced by the brain which influences the kidneys to produce smaller volumes of more concentrated urine.

**atrophy:** Weakening, wasting or degeneration of a tissue — can often be caused by disuse.

**AVP:** Arginine vasopressin, the more modern name for ADH.

**biofeedback:** A form of treatment aimed at helping a person learn to control bodily activities of which she is normally unaware by making information about those activities immediately available.

**bladder training:** A program aimed at gradually increasing the time intervals between urinations and thus increasing the capacity of the bladder.

**BPH:** Benign prostatic hypertrophy, i.e. enlargement of the prostate gland.

**buzzer training:** see pad-and-bell training.

**catheter:** A tube. Catheters used to drain urine are usually passed into the bladder through the urethra but sometimes they are inserted suprapubically i.e. through a small incision in the abdomen above the pubic bone.

**coccyx:** The lowest part of the spine, the tailbone.

**colposuspension:** A commonly-used form of operation for stress incontinence.

**cystitis:** Inflammation of the bladder.

**cystocele:** Bulging of the bladder through the front wall of the vagina.

**cystometry:** A test of bladder function by measuring the amount of liquid the bladder holds and the pressure it produces during filling.

**cystoscopy:** Observation of the inside of the bladder using a type of telescope.

**desmopressin:** A synthetic form of ADH given by nasal spray to treat bedwetting and nocturia.

**detrusor:** The muscle of the bladder which contracts during urination.

# GLOSSARY

**diuresis:** Production of a large volume of urine.

**diuretic:** Promoting diuresis; a substance which encourages increased production of urine.

**dysuria:** Discomfort or pain when passing urine.

**enuresis (nocturnal):** Bedwetting.

**episiotomy:** A cut made in the perineum during childbirth to ease the birth of the baby.

**faradism:** A form of electrical therapy using a single source of fluctuating current.

**fistula:** An abnormal passage or hole e.g. a vesico-vaginal fistula connects the bladder to the vagina and causes continuous dribbling of urine through the vagina.

**flavoxate:** A drug used to treat urge incontinence and related symptoms.

**frequency (urinary):** Urinating seven or more times a day.

**giggle incontinence (giggle micturition):** Involuntary urine loss brought on by extreme giggly laughter.

**haematuria:** The presence of blood in the urine.

**hormone:** A chemical which is produced in one part of the body and circulates in the blood to influence another part, e.g. ADH, oestrogen.

**hypnotherapy:** A treatment using hypnosis.

**hysterectomy:** Surgical removal of the uterus.

**imipramine:** A drug used primarily as an antidepressant but also sometimes used for enuresis. It takes several weeks for the effect to build up.

**incompetence (sphincter):** Inability of the sphincter muscles to close the relevant tube or opening, usually as a result of muscle weakness.

**incontinence (urinary):** The involuntary loss of urine at an inappropriate time or place.

**instability of bladder or detrusor:** The tendency of the bladder muscle in some people to contract inappropriately in response to filling or mild movements.

**interferential therapy:** A form of electrical therapy in which two sources of fluctuating electric current are applied at different points on the body; where they meet deep in the body they 'interfere' with each other and produce an electric field which results in contraction of the muscles.

**levator ani:** The muscles of the pelvic floor which lift the anus when they contract.

**menopause:** The permanent ending of menstrual periods, usually between age 45 and 55, and usually accompanied by other symptoms of the hormonal changes responsible.

**micturition:** Urination, passing water, peeing.

**MSU:** Midstream urine or, loosely, tests carried out on a specimen of urine to check for the presence of e.g. bacteria or blood.

**nocturia:** Needing to wake and empty the bladder at night.

**pad-and-bell training:** A treatment for bedwetting in which a bell or buzzer is used to waken the person if wetness occurs.

**pelvic floor:** The muscles and ligaments at the base of the pelvis which support the internal organs.

**perineometer:** A balloon-like device placed in the vagina to measure the pressure produced by the pelvic floor muscles.

**perineum:** The area between the legs from the anus at the back to the vagina or the base of the penis in front, or more generally the whole 'saddle area' between the legs.

**plication:** Narrowing a hollow organ such as the vagina by stitching tucks or pleats in its walls.

**prolapse:** Loss of normal position of an organ — e.g. the uterus may prolapse and sag into the vagina or, in severe cases, right out of the vagina.

**propantheline:** A drug used to treat urge incontinence and related symptoms.

**prostate gland:** A gland which surrounds the urethra in men and contributes secretions to the semen.

**pubic bone:** The bone at the front of the pelvis, underneath the pubic hair (actually formed from parts of two bones joined in the middle at the pubic symphysis, a joint which normally allows very little movement); see Figure 2 in Chapter 5.

**pubococcygeus:** The major muscle of the pelvic floor, running from the pubic bone to the coccyx; see Figure 3 in Chapter 5.

**rectocele:** Bulging of the rectum through the back wall of the vagina.

**reflex:** An automatic response. The simplest reflexes involve a single sensory nerve and a single responding motor nerve which meet in the spinal cord; complicated reflexes may involve co-ordination between thousands of nerve cells in the brain but they still do not require conscious thought.

**sphincter:** A ring of muscle which controls the opening and closing of a tube (e.g. the urethra) or a body opening (e.g. the anus). Artificial sphincters have been developed for use in cases of severe and intractable incontinence.

**stress incontinence:** Loss of urine with physical stresses which raise the pressure in the abdomen e.g. coughing, sneezing, running, jumping.

**terodiline:** A drug used to treat urge incontinence and related symptoms.

**unstable bladder:** see instability of bladder or detrusor.

**urethra:** The tube which carries urine from the bladder to the outside.

**urethrocele:** Bulging of the urethra into the front of the vagina.

**urge incontinence:** Incontinence preceded by an overwhelming sense of urgency.

**urgency:** The feeling of an urgent need to urinate or of impending urination.

**urodynamics:** Methods for the detailed investigation of the behaviour of the bladder and urethra during filling and emptying.

**uroflowmetry:** Measurement of the rate of flow of urine during bladder emptying.

**uterus:** Womb.

**vasopressin, arginine vasopressin:** ADH.

**voiding difficulty:** Difficulty in emptying the bladder.

# REFERENCES

## References for Chapter 4

1 Beck, RP & Hsu, N (1964) *Am J Obstet Gynecol 89: 820-3* 'Pregnancy, childbirth, and the menopause related to the development of stress incontinence'.

2 Brocklehurst, JC *et al.* (1972) *Age & Ageing 1: 41-7* 'Urinary infections and symptoms of dysuria in women aged 45-64 years: their relevance to similar findings in the elderly'.

3 Bungay, GT, Vessey, MP & McPherson, CK (1980) *Br Med J 281: 181-3* 'Study of symptoms in middle life with special reference to the menopause'.

4 Crist, T, Shingleton, HM & Koch, GG (1972) *Obstet Gynecol 40: 13-7* 'Stress incontinence and the nulliparous patient'.

5 Douglas, JWB (1973) 'Early disturbing events and later enuresis'. In: Kolvin, MacKeith & Meadow (1973)[17] pp 109-17

6 Duncan, AS (1955) *Nursing Mirror 101: (8 April) 10-11* 'Urinary symptoms in obstetrics and gynaecology'.

7 Feneley, RCL *et al.* (1979) *Br J Urol 51: 493-6* 'Urinary Incontinence: prevalence and needs'.

8 Francis, WJA (1960) *J Obstet Gynaec Brit Emp 67: 899-903* 'The onset of stress incontinence'.

9 Glahn, BE (1979) *Br J Urol 51: 363-6* 'Giggle incontinence (enuresis risoria): a study and an aetiological hypothesis'.

10 Glenning, PP (1985) *Aust NZ J Obstet Gynaecol 25: 62-5* 'Urinary voiding patterns of apparently normal women'.

11 Hilton, P (1988) *Br J Obstet Gynaecol 95: 377-81* 'Urinary incontinence during sexual intercourse: a common but rarely volunteered symptom'.

12    Holst, K & Wilson, PD (1988) *New Zealand Medical Journal 101: 756-8* 'The prevalence of female urinary incontinence and reasons for not seeking treatment'.

13    Harding, U *et al.* (1986) *Scand J Urol Nephrol 20: 183-6* 'Urinary incontinence in 45-year-old women: an epidemiological survey'.

14    Iosif, S (1981) *Int J Gynaecol Obstet 19: 13-20* 'Stress incontinence during pregnancy and in puerperium'.

15    Iosif, S, Henriksson, L & Ulmsten, U (1981) *Acta Obstet Gynecol Scand 60: 71-6* 'The frequency of disorders of the lower urinary tract, urinary incontinence in particular, as evaluated by a questionnaire survey in a gynecological health control population'.

16    Jolleys, JV (1988) *Br Med J 296: 1300-2* 'Reported prevalence of urinary incontinence in women in a general practice'.

17    Kolvin, I, MacKeith, R & Meadow, SR (Eds) (1973) *Bladder Control and Enuresis.* London: Heinemann (Clinics in Developmental Medicine **48/49**)

18    Levine, A (1943) *Am J Psychiatry 100: 320-5* 'Enuresis in the Navy'.

19    Low, JA (1964) *Am J Obstet Gynecol 88: 322-35* 'Clinical characteristics of patients with demonstrable urinary incontinence'.

20    Mabeck, CE (1971) *Postgrad Med 47: (suppl) 31-5* 'Uncomplicated urinary tract infection in women'.

21    Mandelstam, D (Ed) (1986) *Incontinence and its Management*, 2nd edn. London: Croom Helm.

22    Nemir, A & Middleton, RP (1954) *Am J Obstet Gynecol 68: 1166-8* 'Stress incontinence in young nulliparous women: a statistical study'.

23    Rees, DLP (1978) *Clinics in Obstet Gynecol 5: 169-92* 'Urinary tract infection'.

24    Rutter, M, Yule, W & Graham, P (1973) 'Enuresis and behavioural deviance: some epidemiological considerations'. In: Kolvin, MacKeith & Meadow (1973)[17] pp137-50

25    Sleep, J & Grant, A (1987) *Br Med J 295: 749-51* 'West Berkshire perineal management trial: three year follow-up'.

26    Sleep, J *et al.* (1984) *Br Med J 289: 587-90* 'West Berkshire perineal management trial'.

27    Sommer, P *et al.* (1990) *Br J Urol 66: 12-15* 'Voiding patterns and prevalence of incontinence in women. A questionnaire survey'.

28    Stanton, SL, Kerr-Wilson, R & Harris, VG (1980) *Br J Obstet Gynaecol 87: 897-900* 'The incidence of urological symptoms in normal pregnancy'.

29    Tchou, DC *et al.* (1988) *Phys Ther 68: 652-5* 'Pelvic-floor musculature exercises in treatment of anatomical urinary stress incontinence'.

30    Thomas, TM *et al.* (1980) *Br Med J 281: 1243-5* 'Prevalence of urinary incontinence'.

31    Thomas, TM (1986) 'The prevalence and health service implications of incontinence,. In: Mandelstam (1986)[21] pp 241-62

32    Thorne, FC (1944) *Am J Psychiatry 100: 686-9* 'Incidence of nocturnal enuresis after age five'.

33  Van Geelen, JM *et al.* (1982) *Am J Obstet Gynecol 144: 636-49* 'The urethral pressure profile in pregnancy and after delivery in healthy nulliparous women'.

34  Walter, S & Olesen, KP (1982) *Br J Obstet Gynaecol 89: 393-401* 'Urinary incontinence and genital prolapse in the female: clinical, urodynamic and radiological investigations'.

35  Wolin, LH (1969) *J Urol 101: 545-9* 'Stress incontinence in young healthy nulliparous female subjects'.

36  Yarnell, JW *et al.* (1981) *J Epidemiol Community Health 35: 71-4* 'The prevalence and severity of urinary incontinence in women'.

# References for Chapter 5

1  Duncan, AS (1955) *Nursing Mirror 101: (8 April) 10-11* 'Urinary symptoms in obstetrics and gynaecology'.

2  Gilpin, SA *et al.* (1989) *Br J Obstet Gynaecol 96: 15-23* 'The pathogenesis of genitourinary prolapse and stress incontinence of urine. A histological and histochemical study'.

3  Jones, EG (1963) *Clinical Obstetrics & Gynecology 6: 220-35* 'Nonoperative treatment of stress incontinence'.

4  Rogers, MP *et al.* (1982) *JAMA 247: 1446-8* 'Giggle incontinence'.

5  Smith, ARB, Hosker, GL & Warrell, DW (1989) *Br J Obstet Gynaecol 96: 24-8* 'The role of partial denervation of the pelvic floor in the aetiology of genitourinary prolapse and stress incontinence of urine. A neurophysiological study'.

6  Smith, ARB, Hosker, GL & Warrell, DW (1989) *Br J Obstet Gynaecol 96: 29-32* 'The role of pudendal nerve damage in the aetiology of genuine stress incontinence in women'.

# References for Chapter 6

1  Godec, CJ (1984) *Urology 23: 97-100* ' "Timed-voiding" — a useful tool in the treatment of urinary incontinence'.

2  James, ED (1978) *Br J Urol 50: 387-94* 'The behaviour of the bladder during physical activity'.

# References for Chapter 7

1  Beck, RP, McCormick, S & Nordstrom, L (1988) *Obstet Gynecol 72: 699-703* 'The fascia lata sling procedure for treating recurrent genuine stress incontinence of urine'.

2  Benvenuti, F *et al.* (1987) *Am J Phys Med 66: 155-68* 'Re-educative treatment of female genuine stress incontinence'.

3  Burgio, KL, Robinson, JC & Engel, BT (1986) *Am J Obstet Gynecol 154: 58-64*

'The role of biofeedback in Kegel exercise training for stress urinary incontinence'.

4   Castleden, CM, Duffin, HM & Mitchell, EP (1984) *Age and Ageing 13: 235-7* 'The effect of physiotherapy on stress incontinence'.

5   Galas, JM *et al*. (1987) *Journal d'Urologie (Paris) 93: 81-6* 'Effects of treatment of female stress incontinence by intravaginal perineal training. Prospective study'. (French with English abstract)

6   Gordon, H & Logue, M (1985) *Lancet ll: (8447, July 20) 123-5* 'Perineal muscle function after childbirth'.

7   Henalla, SM *et al*. (1988) *Br J Obstet Gynaecol 95: 602-6* 'The effect of pelvic floor exercises in the treatment of genuine urinary stress incontinence in women at two hospitals'.

8   Jolleys, JV (1988) *Br Med J 296: 1300-2* 'Reported prevalence of urinary incontinence in women in a general practice'.

9   Jones, EG & Kegel, AH (1952) *Surg Gynecol Obstet 94: 179-88* 'Treatment of urinary stress incontinence with results in 117 patients treated by active exercise of pubococcygei'.

10  Kegel, AH (1948) *Am J Obstet Gynecol 56: 238-48* 'Progressive resistance exercise in the functional restoration of the perineal muscles'.

11  Kegel, AH (1951) *JAMA 146: 915-7* 'Physiologic therapy for urinary stress incontinence'.

12  Low, JA (1967) *Am J Obstet Gynecol 97: 308-15* 'Management of anatomic urinary incontinence by vaginal repair'.

13  Mandelstam, D (1986) 'A programme for re-education'. In: Mandelstam, D (1986)[14] pp 189-194

14  Mandelstam, D (Ed) (1986) *Incontinence and its Management*, 2nd edn. London: Croom Helm

15  Mortensen, S *et al*. (1981) *Prog Clin Biol Res 78: 365-8* 'Long-term results of the abdominal levator ani muscle repair in female urinary incontinence'.

16  Oláh, KS *et al*. (1990) *Am J Obstet Gynecol 162: 87-92* 'The conservative management of patients with symptoms of stress incontinence: a randomized, prospective study comparing weighted vaginal cones and interferential therapy'.

17  Peattie, AB, Plevnik, S & Stanton, SL (1988) *Br J Obstet Gynaecol 95: 1049-53* 'Vaginal cones: a conservative method of treating genuine stress incontinence'.

18  Stanton, SL & Cardozo, LD (1979) *Br J Urol 51: 497-9* 'A comparison of vaginal and suprapubic surgery in the correction of incontinence due to urethral sphincter incompetence'.

19  Stoddart, GD (1983) *Physiotherapy 69: 148-9* 'Research project into the effect of pelvic floor exercises on genuine stress incontinence'.

20  Tchou, DC *et al*. (1988) *Phys Ther 68: 652-5* 'Pelvic-floor musculature exercises in treatment of anatomical urinary stress incontinence'.

21  Wart, F & Roose, G (1984) *Acta Urol Belg 52: 261-8* 'Biofeedback (controlled

auto-relaxation) to complement perineal exercises in the medical treatment of urinary incontinence in women. Preliminary study'. (French with English abstract)

22 Wilson, PD *et al.* (1987) *Br J Obstet Gynaecol 94: 575-82* 'An objective assessment of physiotherapy for female genuine stress incontinence'.

23 Zacharin, RF (1977) *Obstet Gynecol 50: 1-8* 'Abdominoperineal urethral suspension: a ten-year experience in the management of recurrent stress incontinence of urine'.

# References for Chapter 8

1 Cardozo, LD *et al.* (1978) *Br J Urol 50: 521-23* 'Idiopathic bladder instability treated by biofeedback'.

2 Elder, DD & Stephenson, TP (1980) *Br J Urol 52: 467-71* 'An assessment of the Frewen regime in the treatment of detrusor dysfunction in females'.

3 Ferrie, BG *et al.* (1984) *Br J Urol 56: 482-4* 'Experience with bladder training in 65 patients'.

4 Freeman, RM & Baxby, K (1982) *Br Med J 284: 1831-4* 'Hypnotherapy for incontinence caused by the unstable detrusor'.

5 Frewen, WK (1980) *Br J Urol 52: 367-9* 'The management of urgency and frequency of micturition'.

6 Frewen, WK (1982) *Br J Urol 54: 372-3* 'A reassessment of bladder training in detrusor dysfunction in the female'.

7 Frewen, WK (1984) *Br J Urol 56: 330* 'The significance of the psychosomatic factor in urge incontinence'.

8 Holmes, DM *et al.* (1983) *Br J Urol 55: 660-4* 'Bladder training — 3 years on'.

9 Jarvis, GJ & Millar, DR (1980) *Br Med J 281: 1322-3* 'Controlled trial of bladder drill for detrusor instability'.

10 Jeffcoate, TNA & Francis, WJA (1966) *Am J Obstet Gynecol 94: 604-18* 'Urgency incontinence in the female'.

11 Macaulay, AJ *et al.* (1987) *Br Med J 294: 540-3* 'Micturition and the mind: psychological factors in the aetiology and treatment of urinary symptoms in women'.

12 Mahady, IW & Begg, BM (1981) *Br J Obstet Gynaecol 88: 1038-43* 'Long-term symptomatic and cystometric cure of the urge incontinence syndrome using a technique of bladder re-education'.

13 Millard, RJ & Oldenburg, BF (1983) *J Urol 130: 715-9* 'The symptomatic, urodynamic and psychodynamic results of bladder re-education programs'.

14 Pengelly, AW & Booth, CM (1980) *Br J Urol 52: 463-6* 'A prospective trial of bladder training as treatment for detrusor instability'.

15 Sutherst, JR, Brown, MC & Richmond, D (1986) *Br J Urol 58: 273-8* 'Analysis of the pattern of urine loss in women with incontinence as measured by weighing perineal pads'.

16 Svigos, JM & Matthews, CD (1977) *Obstet Gynecol 50: 9-12* 'Assessment and

treatment of female urinary incontinence by cystometrogram and bladder retraining programs'.

# References for Chapter 9

1 Cantor, TJ & Bates, CP (1980) *Br J Obstet Gynaecol 87: 889-92* 'A comparative study of symptoms and objective urodynamic findings in 214 incontinent women'.

2 Edelstein, BA, Keaton-Brasted, C & Burg, MM (1984) *J Consult Clin Psychol 52: 857-62* 'Effects of caffeine withdrawal on nocturnal enuresis, insomnia and behaviour restraints'.

3 Hindmarsh, JR & Byrne, PO (1980) *Br J Urol 52: 88-91* 'Adult enuresis — a symptomatic and urodynamic assessment'.

4 Jarvis, GJ (1982) *Br J Urol 54: 118-9* 'Bladder drill for the treatment of enuresis in adults'.

5 Nørgaard, JP, Pedersen, EB & Djurhuus, JC (1985) *J Urol 134: 1029-31* 'Diurnal anti-diuretic-hormone levels in enuretics'.

6 Torrens, MJ & Collins, CD (1975) *Br J Urol 47: 433-40* 'The urodynamic assessment of adult enuresis'.

# INDEX